COMPUTATIONAL LINGUISTICS IN MEDICINE

IFIP TC-4 Working Conference on
Computational Linguistics in Medicine
Uppsala, Sweden, 2-6 May 1977

Sponsored by
Uppsala University on the occasion of its 500th anniversary
in cooperation with
IFIP Technical Committee 4, Information Processing in Medicine
International Federation for Information Processing

Program Committee:
S. Ohman, A. Pratt, A-L Sagvall Hein
E. Sandewall, W. Schneider, Chairman

NORTH-HOLLAND PUBLISHING COMPANY
AMSTERDAM • NEW YORK • OXFORD

COMPUTATIONAL LINGUISTICS IN MEDICINE

001.5061

**Proceedings of the IFIP Working Conference on
Computational Linguistics in Medicine**

edited by

WERNER SCHNEIDER
and
A-L SÅGVALL HEIN

*Uppsala University Data Center
Uppsala Sweden*

1977

**NORTH-HOLLAND PUBLISHING COMPANY
AMSTERDAM • NEW YORK • OXFORD**

North-Holland ISBN: 0444 85040 6

Published by:
NORTH-HOLLAND PUBLISHING COMPANY
AMSTERDAM • OXFORD • NEW YORK

Distributors for the U.S.A. and Canada:
Elsevier/North-Holland, Inc.
52 Vanderbilt Avenue
New York, N.Y. 10017

PRINTED IN THE NETHERLANDS

PREFACE

The aim of this working conference was to study how and to what extent the application of methods from computational linguistics (CL) and artificial intelligence (AI) can contribute to the automatic processing of verbal medical information and to the modelling of medical knowledge and medical decision processes.

The conference was organized into three parts. The first part was centered around certain issues in computational linguistics and artificial intelligence, relevant to medical applications. This part served as a theoretical framework for the rest of the conference. It was also intended as a stimulus to the introduction of new approaches into the field. Part two was devoted to medical systems and applications, involving verbal information processing. Part three, finally, was focussed on implementation aspects and requirements on hardware and software.

It was considered most important to give the speakers ample time for presentations and detailed discussions. In addition, demonstrations of the following systems were arranged: The Medical Information Processing System at NIH, Pratt, Bethesda; UCLA Natural Language Retrieval System, Lamson, Los Angeles; MYCIN, Shortliffe, Stanford; The Present Illness System, Pauker, Boston; CONDOR, Banerjee, Munich; COMPADOS, van Egmond, Gent; LIsp DAta base Manager, Risch, Uppsala. These demonstrations were all successful (!!) which substantially enhanced the understanding of the different contributions to the conference.

Two topics were brought up for general discussion: problems concerning special requirements on hardware and software and the impact of CL and AI on medicine.

The conference demonstrated the great power of the new technology discussed. CL and AI techniques will certainly have great impact on medicine, especially on education and clinical decision-making. We are, however, still at the very beginning and much research and development has to be performed before clinical practice may directly benefit. What concerns education, the conference made it clear that significant achievments can be made already within the next few years.
Thus, we are convinced that this field is one of those which really deserves all possible support. This is a challenge for the future to all those who are involved in the field of information processing in medicine.

We want to express our sincere thanks to Uppsala University, especially to the Rector Magnificus, Prof T Segerstedt and to the Executive Vice-President, Dr G Wijkman for having sponsored this symposium. Very special thanks go to Kerstin Sjöberg who did so much for the detailed organization of the meeting as well as for the preparation of the proceedings. We gratefully acknowledge the extensive work invested by those who made all the successful demonstrations possible, especially Carl Cederlund, IBM Medical Industry Center, Stockholm, Gunnar Hårdsten, SAAB/UNIVAC, Stockholm, Donna Taeuber and Dr Banerjee, SIEMENS AG, Munich and their collaborators from SIEMENS AG, Sweden, Ruby Okubo, UCLA, Scotty Carlisle and Dr Rindfleish, Stanford, Tore Risch and Sven G Johansson, Uppsala. We are especially indebted to Hans-Åke Ramdén, Uppsala, who was the coordinator of all these demonstrations.

What would a meeting be without a banquet? Thank you IBM Medical Industry Center, especially Lennart Naroskin and Carl Cederlund for a wonderful evening.

Finally, we want to thank Jan Roukens, the chairman of IFIP-TC4, for his kind
support of the meeting and Stephanie Smit and Dr Einar Fredriksson from North
Holland Publishing Company and Dr Stellan Bengtsson from Uppsala University for
their invaluable assistance in editing and publishing these proceedings.
For readers who feel unfamiliar with concepts and notions used in this book we
have included a list of references to some of the most important basic literature
in the fields covered.

Uppsala in May 1977

Anna-Lena Sågvall
Werner Schneider

Uppsala University Datacenter (UDAC)

TABLE OF CONTENTS

WELCOMING ADDRESS
by
Dr. Gunnar Wijkman
Executive vice-president of Uppsala University

On behalf of Uppsala University I wish you heartily welcome to this Symposium on Computational Linguistics in Medicine. For us it is a pleasure and an honour that so many have responded to our invitation. This Symposium is part of a series of about 50, by which the University wants to celebrate its 500 year Jubilee.

It has been our ambition, in the planning of this Jubilee, to make it not only a traditional celebration with some days of special festivities, but also - and perhaps we consider that as more important - an encouragement and a support to the scientists and the staff of our University. We want to make use of the Jubilee, taking advantage of the fact that prominent scientists from the whole world would probably be more interested in coming to Uppsala in such a year. It seems today that we are right on that point.

A main thought in our planning of the Symposia has been that we should not rest on our laurels but look ahead and let this year initiate a new series of active years - why not another 500?
Thus, we hope that the main theme of each Symposium would be the scientific guideline for the next years to come and also a vision of towards what aims and in what direction Science is developing.

In connection with the Jubilee we have also tried to document what has been done and what constitutes science in Uppsala today. Thus each Faculty has published a volume describing the development in its different sections and what they are dealing with today, in all seventeen volumes. In many cases they have tried to consider the question of what the future will look like. These publications and the reports from the Symposia ought to form an interesting historical documentation and a report on what is done scientifically in Uppsala in 1977, how we considered the future development and, finally, how the foreign Symposia participants looked at it. Then it remains to guess when this information will be of interest - in 10 or in 100 or in 500 years. Perhaps it will be of special interest to see how the development will correspond to the prognoses in 1977 here in Uppsala.

It is probable that this symposium on Computational Linguistics in Medicine will be of special interest from the points of view mentioned earlier since in this field we have to look forward to a very fast development in the near future. In a longrange perspective computational linguistics and artificial intelligence techniques will perhaps introduce a basic and interesting change concerning storing and processing of information.

I remember with pleasure a report, presented at a congress on hospital administration in Zagreb some years ago. What I found most fascinating was the use of systems analysis applied to a complicated information process. On the basis of such thorough analyses, the computer could be used where it could be most effective under the given conditions.

What strikes you as an amateur in this area is that we still are, to a great extent, forced to adapt to the requirements of the computer. Perhaps this is most accentuated in administration where we had to adapt to a formalized input and communication procedure as well as to an extensive control that we are "understood" by the computer instead of using our "real-time" manual information processing. Today we can rapidly get the information the different systems are designed to produce, but if we want an alternative use of the stored information e.g. a general survey, the work becomes so complicated that we have to give up.

Sometimes, when you have to ask a technician to produce the material, you long for the old solid card system.

I hope and expect that development in the field of artificial intelligence and computational linguistics will soon make it possible to process stored information in several ways without time-consuming and costly reprogramming.

In this area as in all areas the computer systems have come to stay. I believe that, after all, we stand at the beginning of a period of development. We shall have new possibilities to collect and systematize information, and much better possibilities to interpret it than we could ever imagine. We shall be able to select the information and make it as easily accessible as the books in our bookshelves.

It is not unlikely that, in the future, people will talk about our times with regard to the computer area in the same way as we talk today of the time when the art of printing took its first stumbling steps.

I am convinced that this Symposium will actively contribute to the development in the computer area and I wish you good luck.

WELCOMING ADDRESS
by
Jan Roukens
Chairman of IFIP-TC4

Doctor Wijkman, dear host. Your belief in today's subject and your ability to convince have made this conference possible. It is a great pleasure for me, and a great honour for the International Federation for Information Processing, to be allowed to take part in the celebration of that act of foresightedness, 500 years ago, which created the world-famous university of Uppsala. I hope that this scientific meeting will give us more knowledge about the basic requirements for better communication in medical practice, research and education, and that it will remain a sparkling piece in the chain of events that form the spiritual history of this University;

Werner Schneider, to few people IFIP-TC4 owes so much. This is not your last enterprise in 1977. The baroque variation of your ideas, expressions and gestures, is guided by a disciplined social conscience. This has lead you, among other things, to organizing this Working Conference on Computational Linguistics and Artificial Intelligence in Medicine together with Anna-Lena Sågvall Hein;

Dear Anna-Lena on behalf of TC4 my sincere thanks for the heavy burden of all the work you have done in the Organizing and Program Committees and for the editing of the Proceedings of this conference;

Dear friends, speakers and discussants:

A very warm welcome to you all on behalf of the IFIP Committee for Health Care and Biomedical Research (TC4).

As an introduction to some personal comments on the subject of this conference, let me quote our godfather Wittgenstein, who offered me the following fundamental remark (Philosophical Investigations, I, 292): "Glaub nicht immer, dass du deine Worte von Tatsachen abliest, diese nach Regeln in Worte abbildest! Denn die Anwendung der Regel im besonderen Fall müsstest du ja doch ohne Führung machen".
In English:
"Don't think that you can read off what you say from the facts; that you portray the facts in words according to rules. Because even if such a rule would exist, the application of it in a particular case has to be done by you without guidance".

Computational Linguistics in Medicine is a different field than Medical Linguistics. I understand that the Program Committee has intentionally chosen the title as it stands. Whereas Medical Linguistics is the science that deals with the language spoken and written in medical circles, computational linguistics deals with (written) language elements as data, to which algorithms can be applied. Language is then defined as letters and punctuation marks and spaces, then words, sentences, paragraphs or chapters, and so on. Some only partially known rules to describe how to compose the higher order from the lower order elements are also included. A most elementary form of Computational Linguistics is simple counting. I quote James T. MacDonough, who stated in a 1961 symposium on computers and literature:
"The Iliad is a narrative poem. More specifically, it has about 112,000 words, arranged in 15,694 dactylic hexameter lines....."
The more sophisticated forms of Computational Linguistics seem to deal with the transformations of natural languages into each other, or with semantic feature extraction which maps natural language forms onto an artificial language. The experiences gained with these extremely speculative areas of Computational Linguistics have not been very encouraging. The reason is, that algorithms transforming natural language strings into each other do not exist. In order to trans-

late it is necessary to extract the semantic content of a written expression, and express this again in the other language.

The problem of selective retrieval of natural language texts, often referred to as information retrieval, is of intermediate complexity. The relative simplicity of the problem can be illustrated superficially with the hunting of ducks or similar birds. After each loosely directed shot with a multitude of small bullets, some ducks will fall down. And if one is not satisfied with the number brought down, another shot may be tried for more. The shooting can be done by the system, but with information retrieval the eating is left to man.

To me a most important field of research in medicine seems to be the investigation of the feasibility of constructing artificial languages, of which the basic elements are the medical nomenclatures. Strictly speaking, the creation of artificial languages in medicine is part of the science of Medical Linguistics: which is a lot of medicine and some linguistics. Simple computational procedures may be of great help, though, with the creation of artificial systematized nomenclatures. In my opinion a main goal for this conference is a critical evaluation of what is worth-while and what is false or without sense in the fields of computational and medical linguistics. There is no doubt that the mediocre effectiveness and efficiency of information exchange in medical practice, medical research and medical education is a constant threat to the effectiveness and efficiency of our health care system as a whole. We should try to analyze the different attempts for solutions that are proposed, and decide which are worth-while to pursue and which are not.

The problems apparent in medicine in the areas of information transfer, decision making and problem solving, problems with which this conference will be dealing, are too important to be obscured by vague thinking.

I hope that this meeting be sharp as a lancet in cutting away all that obscures the problems we are faced with; let the conference clarify the strategies and methods that solve the problems under consideration.

Thank you.

PART I

METHODOLOGICAL BACKGROUND

Computational Linguistics in Medicine, Schneider/Sagvall Hein, eds.
North-Holland Publishing Company, (1977)

THE IMPACT OF CL AND AI TECHNIQUES ON MODELLING IN MEDICINE

Werner Schneider
Uppsala University Data Center, Uppsala, Sweden

At the beginning of the 1970's an increasing number of people came to the conclusion that the first decade of computer usage in the field of health care was essentially an era of over-promises and under-achievements. However, in spite of all the disappointments and frustrations, most of them were still convinced that computer techniques - properly developed and applied - will lead to significant improvements in health care delivery. One of them was the head of the university hospital in Uppsala, Prof. Anders Grönwall. During his presidency of the International Hospital Federation (IHF) he proposed late in 1973 - as one of the steps to be taken in the course of recovery and reorientation - the formation of an international study group for the purpose of preparing a report, describing the state-of-the-art concerning the application of computer techniques in health care with special regard to hospitals. The group was formed and the report it prepared was presented and discussed at the IHF congress in Zagreb in 1975. Let me comment briefly on just some of the points and conclusions made in this report (1), because they have, as a matter of fact, lead to the organization of this meeting. The report reveals that the successful usage of computer techniques in health care is restricted almost exclusively to a few well-defined areas in administration and to some medical services such as fiscal accounting and some types of laboratory automation. Expressed in more technical terms the report stated that computer usage was successful in those cases where
(1) the existing and/or envisaged processing of information was clearly defined and explicitly describable
(2) the character of the processing of information involved was of the numerical and/or the bit/byte/field-shuffling type and
(3) the processing of information inherent to a subsystem of activities within the health care system was computerized without unbalancing the subsystem as such or its interactions with other subsystems as defined by the overall system.

Conditions (1) and (2) merely reflect the fact that the basic construction of hardware and software has not essentially changed since the first computers were invented for solving ballistic problems in World War II and for further mechanization in the area of commercial business as e.g. billing and advertising procedures. They restrict computer usage in health care as mentioned above to very dedicated areas such as
- laboratories as e.g. clinical chemical laboratories, where a large number of relatively simple numerical calculations has to be per formed in combination with manyfold reporting procedures involvingextensive byte- and field-shuffling, or radiophysics departments, where the calculation of appropriate irradiation dosages requires advanced number crunching.
- intensive care units where a large number of more or less advanced numerical calculations have to be performed in real time and where at the same time very advanced byte- and field-shuffling is required for real-time reporting of results in a number of alphanumeric or graphic displays.
- administrative units in the health care system, where mainly processing of the bit/byte/field-shuffling type is required, as is the case in fiscal accounting routines, tabulations, and health screening procedures for groups of individuals etc.

The third condition implicates limitations concerning the introduction of computer techniques even in those areas where they are adequate from the technical point of view. It merely requires a systems analysis of the subsystem of activities within the health care system in which computerized information processing is

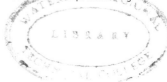

envisaged prior to the development and implementation of the computerized procedures. This is, however, a very difficult task because of the fact that the
degree of complexity of the activity pattern of even small and limited functional
units is in most cases beyond that which can be treated by standard methods of
operations research. The highly dynamic character of the various subsystems of
the health care system is in general the real "point de résistance". Only during
the last few years have more powerful - computer based - techniques been developed
which make more appropriate systems analysis in the area of health care possible
(see e.g. (2)). The previous lack of this kind of methodology explains the fact
that computer usage has often been unsuccessful even in those areas where success
was possible from the point of view of adequacy of the available hardware and
software. We are, however, even here still at the very beginning (3). As we will
see later on in this paper the basic problems met in the area of analysis and
evaluation of existing and planned subsystems and their interaction with other
subsystems within the health care system are of the same nature as those we
struggle with when attempting to use computer techniques in clinical medicine:
The lack of formalized knowledge and adequate techniques for accomplishing
formalization of knowledge in the various fields of medicine. Although omission
of systems analysis prior to the introduction of computers into laboratories,
intensive care units and different areas of health care administration caused
much frustration in many places, the loss of money involved was still reasonably
low. The situation was much worse in those cases where computers were introduced
to areas in health care, where none of the three conditions mentioned above was
fulfilled. This happened mostly in the various fields of medical care, especially
remedial care in hospitals. The logical conclusion would have been that the
first thing to do was to concentrate any available resources on efforts to
formalize the existing knowledge concerning the highly dynamic processes in the
human biological and behavioral system on one hand and in the health care system
on the other hand, including the creation of adequate formalizing techniques.
Unfortunately only a few understood that it is exactly here where computer
technology will play its most important role (see e.g. (4)).
For many reasons the majority of people involved in medical computing did not
draw this conclusion. The strategy adopted instead was to adapt medicine as far
as possible to fit existing computerized information processing methodology as
it is used by statisticians and in the field of natural science. The basic idea
was that more data - especially more so-called "hard"-data, i.e. measured by
natural science methodology - would produce more and better information and that
more information would lead to better decisions. As a consequence a large number
of sometimes huge databanks have been established, mostly based on a rather
random choice of which data should be collected and treated by more or less
advanced statistical procedures. This approach is of course fundamentally wrong.
It is still, however, the most commonly used approach in spite of all the frustrations it already accounts for. There are many reasons for that, one is the
decreasing cost of disc storage devices, another the availability of commercial
database handling software and still another an easily made and widely spread
misunderstanding of Shannon's theory of communication (see (5)).
Obviously only those data which are relevant for the description of the processes
under consideration are of importance. This selection can, however, in most cases
not be made at all, because of the fact that there are no cues available, which
would provide for an appropriate linkage between the data stored in the databank
and the processes they are emanating from. The omission of preserving these cues
causes a fundamental loss of information, which can not be repaired by any statistical method. But even in the case where the relevance of data to a specific
context can be judged we are confronted with the problem of their relative importance for an adequate description of the processes they are related to. This
evaluation can only be made on the basis of an adequate formalized description of
the process under consideration. One of the basic reasons for theory formation is
as a matter of fact to determine the relevance of different observations in the
context of a specific problem. To try to compensate the lack of knowledge - due
to the absence of an adequate formalized description - concerning the intrinsic

relations between observations - data - on a specific process by collecting more
data is doomed to fail. The fundamental loss of information is of the same
nature as discussed above and cannot be repaired by any statistical method. That
more data do not necessarily create more and better information and that more
information does not necessarily lead to better decisions is clear to anybody
who has tried to make better conclusions out of a picture in a newspaper by
applying a magnifying glass. However, until now, the theoretical background in
terms of a well developed theory of information has been lacking. Still only few
scientists are tackling the problem. Recently made progress in this respect
seems, however, to be most promising for the future (see e.g. (6)).
In the absence of these improvements we will, unfortunately, still for many
years be confronted with sales pressures from medical industries and computer
manufacturers who want us to buy more and more advanced technical equipment,
measuring in any detail any kind of continuous or discontinuous signals, analyzing
them by the most powerful mathematical and statistical methods, consuming extensive computer resources, producing any kind of data which are in no significant
relation to the decision process in health care. Names as Fourier and Walsh are
almost equivalent to those of religious prophets in the era of computer salvation.
There are of course many other aspects to the problem "data - information -
knowledge - decision" which might be discussed in this connexion. In the context
of this paper it is important to discuss just one more in further detail. Both
the - biological and behavioral - system called "human being" and the health
care system consist of a huge number of highly dynamic processes. Obviously the
techniques for the description of these processes must be adapted to these
fundamental characteristics. Unfortunately it is here we meet the real difficulties mainly because of the lack of adequate formalization techniques. Naturally
many basic mistakes were made when trying to go around these difficulties. Again
one believed - and many people still do - that the availability of more data was
a good way to do so. A typical approach, still widely used and tried in this
sense, is the so-called pattern recognition approach. The most usual mistake
made when using this approach is the following: One assumes that, measuring a
large amount of data concerning a specific system at a specific point of time
allows for highly significant predictions and conclusions if this pattern is
compared with a large number of similar patterns of similar systems which are
stored in a huge databank. This is of course true, however, only under very
specific and well defined circumstances which in the dynamic environment of
health care can rarely be arranged; but even in those cases no real insight
concerning the processes involved is gained by this methodology. The scope of
this paper limits us to discuss only the probably most severe restriction to
this approach. There is, from the mathematical point of view just one situation
where "success" is certain: The systems behaviour must fulfill the requirements
of an analytic function and all derivatives must be known in the point where the
"pattern" is to be determined. Obviously in an environment of multiple multidimen-
sional dynamic processes this is not possible. According to this approach the
established databanks are therefore merely highly expensive data cemeteries. The
IHF study group has summarized the problem discussed until now as follows:
"Is it possible or indeed desirable to include all possible data in a computer
data base with the hope that some later retrospective search and retrieval will
require or even use these data? This approach is now recognized as one ardently
to be avoided! The dynamic nature and the changing processes in care affected by
scientific and technical development at the same time make definition of a uni-
form general data base difficult at best. Poorly defined problems create major
difficulties in defining data bases containing information which will provide
desired answers. The uncertain quality and insufficiency of the available data
were often given less attention than creating elegant algorithms. The variable
and often closely circumscribed relevance and adequacy of available algorithms
provided inadequate answers, for example, in terms of patient care decision
support. Far more emphasis was placed on the mechanism for generating answers
than on formulating pertinent questions. All of these situations strongly suggest
that a comprehensive large-scale mass storage of data as the initial effort in

ADP application in the hospital is likely to be futile. Such an approach merges assorted and unspecified semantic and contextually dependent data bases. These data include terms or descriptors often without appropriate related values or quantities or time relationships."
At the end of the IHF congress in Zagreb 1975 the executive vice-president of Uppsala University, Dr. Gunnar Wijkman, asked some of the study group the follow- ing question: Although I appreciate all the good advices you have laid down in your report on how we can smoothly accomplish a more efficient and meaningful usage of computers in hospitals and health care I would like to know: In what fields of research and development would you invest your money if you in a long- term perspective of a few decades wanted to make sure that essential progress in health care is achieved? There was full agreement on a few topics; one of the most important was the formalization of knowledge concerning the highly dynamic processes in the human biological system on one hand and in the health care system on the other hand, including the creation of adequate formalizing techni- ques". Dr. Wijkman proposed as a consequence of this discussion to sponsor a brain storming symposium on this topic in the frame of the scientific program, devoted to the celebration of the 500th anniversary of the Uppsala University. Who could resist such a challenging offer? Now we are here, and we will hopefully make a good start for important future research and development in a field which we believe to be even more important now than we did two years ago in Zagreb. One among us is probably especially happy about the realization of this meeting: Prof. Francois Grémy who already on a fine, warm summer day in Stockholm in 1974 suggested that I organize a TC4 Working Conference on Computational Linguistics in Medicine in Uppsala.

How does the theme of the conference relate to the more general description of "what should be done" as presented to Dr. Wijkman?
It is often emphasized that medicine x) is not only a science but also an art. We can reformulate this statement in technical terms as follows:
That part of medical knowledge which already is explicitly formulated constitutes the science called medicine. That part which still only is available in implicit form constitutes the art called medicine. Implicitly formulated medical knowledge is sometimes exclusively "implemented" in the brain of one single expert, some- times it is available in extensive verbal descriptions. Communication of this knowledge is very unsatisfactory, it is many times limited to audiovisual means. As a consequence, education of medical students and health care staff is sometimes very poor and still allows for "prophets" and "schools" bearing the names of them. Why is in the field of medicine, especially in the area of mental diseases, still the largest portion of knowledge not explicitly formulated? The reason lies clearly in the absence of adequate formalizing techniques. Whereas in most fields of the natural sciences, mathematics with all its different specialities was and still to large extent is sufficient for the purpose of explicit formalization, this is only true for a very restricted part of medicine. Still even in the pro- bably most formalized experimental field of natural science, physics, the problem of formalizing knowledge is an issue of greatest importance. Therefore many dis- tinguished physicists have dealt extensively with it. In the context of this pa- per I think it is interesting to cite especially two of them: the late Nobel-Price winner Wolfgang Pauli stated many years ago that o) "Through the fact that modern psychology proves that any kind of understanding is a tedious process which is initiated through processes of the unconscious a long time before a rational for- malization of contents of the conscious can take place, attention has been re- directed to the preconscious and archaic level of cognition. Instead of clear

---

x) Here and in the sequel clinical psychology is included in the term medicine. It is beyond the scope of this paper to discuss this definition in more detail. Let us just state that "hardware" and software" can be distinguished in a human being although they can interact strongly, as is the case in much simpler sys- tems, as for example digital computers.
o) Translated from German.

concepts there exist, on this level, images with strong emotional contents which
are not "thought" but "viewed in painting"" (see (7)). Depending on the state
and the complexity of such an understanding process different techniques can be
used to explicitly formulate what has been understood up to this point for
external and/or internal communication. There is a difficult choice to be made
between a variety of such techniques: plain natural language, special scientific
dialects of natural language, artificial languages, logic, mathematics, etc.
etc. The late Nobel-Price winner Werner Heisenberg (8) commented about logic and
natural language as follows: x) "In the domain of logic, attention is focused on
special linguistic structures, on anambiguous connexions between assumptions and
conclusions, on simple models of inference; all other linguistic structures are
disregarded. These other structures consist e.g. of associations between certain
secondary meanings of words; a secondary meaning of a word, which is, so to
speak, just gliding through the twilight of the conscious, when the word is
pronounced, still may contribute essentially to the content of a sentence. The
fact that every word can cause many, only semi-consciuous, movements in our
thinking implies that natural language can be used for representing certain
aspects of reality in a more distinctive manner than it would be possible with
the aid of logic inference procedures." Unfortunately there is a considerable
gap between natural language on one hand and the languages of logic, mathematics
etc. on the other hand. Therefore many scientists especially in the field of
medicine would like to have "something in between", i.e. some kind of more
advanced and more flexible modelling techniques. o) Consider for illustration
the following examples:
A very restricted but still very interesting area of biomedical research is the
study of iron-kinetics in man. One of the basic experimental techniques used in
this field is to observe the behaviour of intravenously injected radioiron in
plasma and the red cells. On the basis of such experimental data and a lot of
other experimental and theoretical knowledge available concerning the different
biomedical processes in which iron in the human body is involved, a group of
scientists in Uppsala including myself started about 17 years ago to tackle the
problem of further formalizing knowledge in this area. The first step in this
course of "theory-formation" in the field of iron-kinetics of man was a rather
simple model (11) which still could be formulated mathematically in terms of
analytically solvable differential equations, even though programmable electronic
calculators are needed for a detailed interpretation of the analytically formulated result. This model was, however, not compatible with some medical knowledge
especially concerning the bone marrow part in it (12). Thus more sophisticated
mechanisms had to be included representing the maturation of and the iron uptake
by red cell precursors in the bone marrow as well as the premature death of newly
formed red cells. Although it was still possible to formulate these extended
models in terms of differential equations it was not longer possible to solve
them analytically. It even turned out that these systems of differential equations
were not easily treated by standard computer based methods of numerical integration (13). Because experimenting with different model structures thus became
rather soon cumbersome we looked for other formalizing techniques, and I still
remember when I introduced the notions of "simulation models" and "computer
simulation" to my colleagues from the field of biomedicine. As a matter of fact
the modelling process was significantly enhanced by reformulating the context in
terms of a simulation model and experimenting with the aid of simulation techniques although it was not necessary from the strict point of view of formalizing
knowledge. We even suggested not to use simulation techniques as soon as a model
should for any reason reach a rather permanent status (13). Clearly these models

---

x) Translated from German
o) There exist of course many definitions of the terms "modelling" and "models".
One of the most important is probably Tarski's definition in the context of
formalized theories (9). In this paper, however, modelling is defined as being
that major component in theory formation, which accomplishes the transition from
implicit to explicit knowledge. A more formal and thorough analysis of the process
of theory formation will be presented in a forthcoming paper (10).

are borderline cases and they are therefore, of course especially interesting in
the frame work of investigations concerning the power and limits of various
formalizing techniques (14).
It is very easy to understand that rather simple conceptual extensions of the
model of ironkinetics in man discussed here would exclude "simpler" approaches
than simulation techniques. In clinical psychology this is almost always the
case. When Prof. Ulrich Moser (he will attend the second part of this meeting),
Dr. Ilka von Zeppelin and myself reported on our common research project concerning computer simulation of a model of neurotic defence mechanisms we commented
the issue of formalization in the following way (see (15) pages 53 and 54; see
also (16) and (17) page 194): "All formalization is concerned with the development
of concepts. It takes as its starting-point experimental data or clinical observations. The verification or falsification of concepts (the sum total of which can
be called a theory) can again only take effect of the basis of empirical scrutiny.
Formalization consists in the search for suitable and specific languages. If we
consider metapsychological concepts, for example, we notice that they are to a
high degree accompanied by purely verbal connotative meanings which make it
difficult to formulate relations with clarity. The aim we set ourselves was to
formulate a restricted area of metapsychology in non-verbal concepts. We did not
go so far as a mathematical formulation of psychic processes (in the form of
differential equations), but we employed the less strict form of an algorithm,
formulated in a computer language.
There were good grounds for making this attempt, and it was not by chance that
the mechanisms of defence were chosen as the point of departure. Psychoanalytic
thinking lays claim to exact attention to psychodynamic processes and genetic
structuration. Metapsychological concepts are, however, still not sufficiently
differentiated to make such formalization really possible. In the theory of the
defence mechanisms a distinction is made between various defence techniques
(repression, identification, projection, regression, etc.) without it being
possible to effect exact formalization of the circumstances and time sequence.
The defence techniques come into play in a neurotic conflict. Strict formalization
increases the possibility of establishing functional connections between the
variables, and in this manner the concepts are functionally defined in a model.
They can no longer, as in the case of verbal theories, be employed differently
in various contexts. In the course of our work it became clear that, owing to
the process of formalization, some metapsychological concepts would have to be
newly defined. It would not be correct, however, to speak of "neologisms". The
attempt to apply our model to clinical situations will immediately make clear
why it was imperative to effect modifications.
The formalization process leads to a temporary structuration in a model. This
has the advantage of enabling clear formulation of hypotheses which can be
falsified through empirical experience. It is thus likely that certain assumptions
in the model (e.g. the assumptions of the hierarchic and genetic arrangement of
the defence mechanisms), concerning which no exact empirical findings exist,
will turn out to be false. However, in psychoanalysis too we shall have to
become accustomed to employing falsification methods instead of a procedure
which seeks confirmatory evidence for a hypothesis.
The formalization of concepts is a continuous process. There is no final model,
just as there is no model which is of absolute validity."
In the field of clinical psychology as well as in general clinical medicine even
the use of mathematically formulated simulation models is, however, limited. As a
matter of fact it seems that the use of this kind of technique is restricted to
the representation of control- and monitor-structures of dynamic systems in these
fields. Although such models represent a major step forward in the process of
theory formation in psychology (18) there is still a malaise among psychologists
concerning the question whether or not to prefer to formalize knowledge verbally.
This reflects of course rather well the borderline area described by Heisenberg
and it has at this point become clear that it is in this domain real innovation
is required. Through many years it has been my persuasion that the various research
projects which run under the badly, but for our purpose sufficiently well defined
name "artificial intelligence" on the one hand and research in computational

linguistics on the other hand will be the main contributors of insight and instru-
mentation needed for accomplishing the progress concerning techniques for formalizing knowledge we are looking for. To avoid any misunderstanding let me reformulate this statement in the following way: AI and CL will not solve our problems
in medicine. Progress in these fields results, however, in spin-offs which are
prerequisites for real innovational steps on the way to better understand and
formally describe the human biological system as well as the health care systems.
x) Examples of such spin-offs are the availability of programming systems as
LISP, KRL-0, as well as of advanced parsing systems etc.

The impact of these new computer techniques is clearly revealed by many of the
contributions to this seminar. We are, of course, still at the very beginning.
Dynamic problems e.g., can at the moment hardly be tackled by available AI-
techniques.
The extension of LISP to SLISP (19) implying that the main facilities of the
widely used simulation language SIMULA now are available in a LISP-environment
(e.g. LISP 1.6 or INTERLISP), is a most interesting step forward in this respect.
A major attempt to tackle the problem of representing knowledge about complex
dynamic systems, with special regard to cognitive processes, is made in PSYPAC.
It will be presented during this conference.
We could conclude here and just look forward to a time when the major part of
medicine is a science and only a minor part still can be called an art, trusting
the fact that formalizing of medical knowledge will progress rapidly because of
an increasing number of important spin-offs from CL and AI becoming available.
Unfortunately we would then still not have done very much for the clinician in
his every-day practice. Why?
In clinical practice the main problem is to interprete observations about a
progressing illness or disability in a human being in terms of existing medical
knowledge, in a first approach of the medical knowledge immediately available to
the specific responsible doctor. This process of interpretation is extremely
complex. Among other things it comprises a simultaneous real-time simulation of
all those models available in the actual human knowledge base, which describe
processes which could possibly be the ones really going on in the patient. Matching and evaluation is repeatedly done as a function of time implying among other
things that some of the models have to be re-run a few times, in order to find
out under what conditions of malfunctioning of the processes they describe, a
match with observed data can be obtained. To improve present, brain based clinical information processing and decision making by computer techniques is obviously extremely difficult. A prerequisite is evidently that a computerized knowledge
base includes representations of more or less complex dynamic processes and
systems. A most interesting approach to assist the kind of information processing,
going on in clinical practice, by AI and CL techniques has been made in a completely different field, i.e. electronics, by Brown and Burton from BBN (20). Of
course their system, called SOPHIE, cannot be transplanted directly to the field
of clinical medicine. It is, however, of great interest from different points of
view, as e.g. its structure, its representation of knowledge about dynamic processes, its self-explanatory facilities, its processing of natural language etc.
etc. The importance of the availability of adequate self-explanatory facilities
in this kind of CL and AI based systems, we are looking for, can not be overempha-
sized. The MYCIN system, which will be presented during this symposium, is for
the moment being probably the leading one in this respect.
Systems as SOPHIE and the one which will be presented by Dr. Pauker in this
symposium clearly demonstrate the severe limitations of the Bayesian approach.
Fortunately for the patients, clinicians are not Bayesian machines, disregarding
the dynamics of the human biological and behavioral systems.

Let me finally comment about a technical problem concerning the use of more and
more developed computerized knowledge databases. The fact that they can only be

---

x) This is even true for such projects which deal with the creation of artificial
medical languages based e.g. on existing medical nomenclatures.

implemented in languages which are fully incompatible with the software normally used for databases represents a major difficulty. The DATAMANAGER presented by Prof. Sauter and demonstrated by Dr. Risch during this symposium is a major attempt to overcome this difficulty: Extending the present version by stepwise implementing knowledge bases and CL techniques is easily done as long as they are written in LISP, the most used programming language in this field.

REFERENCES

(1) W. Schneider and S. Bengtsson, eds: The Application of Computer Techniques in Health Care, Comp. Progr. Biomed. 5 (1975), 171-249.
(2) B. Sandblad: Systems Analysis and Simulation of Health Care Laboratory Systems: Acta Universitatis Upsaliensis 420, Almquist & Wiksell Int., Stockholm 1977.
(3) B. Sandblad, W. Schneider and W.A. Spencer: Modelling Techniques for Analysis of the External Effectiveness of Health Care Laboratory Functions, Technical report UPTEC 77 17 R, Inst. of Technology, Uppsala University, 1977. To be published in Medical Informatics.
(4) W. Schneider: Development of Advanced Database Software Techniques, Proc. of MEDIS'73, Osaka, Kansai Inst. of Inf. Systems, 1973.
(5) C.E. Shannon and W. Waever: The Mathematical Theory of Communication, Bell System Tech. J. 27, 1948.
(6) L. Preuss: A Primer of Information Dynamics, Internal Report, Infodyn Inc., Zürich and Uppsala University Datacenter, Uppsala, 1975.
(7) W. Pauli: Einfluss archetypischer Vorstellungen auf die Bildung naturwissenschaftlicher Theorien bei Kepler, in: C.G. Jung and W. Pauli: Naturerklärung und Psyche, 109-194, Zürich, 1952.
(8) W. Heisenberg: Physik und Philosophie, Weltperspektiven, Vol. 2, Ullstein GmbH Verlag, Frankfurt a/M, 1959.
(9) A. Tarski: Logic, Semantics and Metamathematics, page 416, Oxford Univ. Press, 1953.
(10) W. Schneider: Some aspects on theory formation, to be published in Comp. Progr. Biomed.
(11) L. Garby, W. Schneider, O. Sundquist and J.C. Vuille, Acta Physiol. Scand., 59, Suppl. 216 (1963).
(12) J.C. Vuille, Acta Physiol, Scand., 65, Suppl. 253 (1965), 3.
(13) T. Groth, W. Schneider, E. Sandewall and J.C. Vuille, Computer Simulation of Ferrokinetic Models, Comp. Progr. Biomed. 1 (1970), 90-104.
(14) R. Pfeifer and W. Schneider: Modelling and formalizing languages, in preparation.
(15) U. Moser, I. v Zeppelin and W. Schneider, Computer Simulation of a Model of Neurotic Defence Processes, Int. J. of Psycho-Analysis, 50 (1969), 53-64.
(16) U. Moser, W. Schneider and I. v Zeppelin, Ueber den Wert der Computersimulation in der Neurosenforschung, Schweiz. Zeitschr. f. Psychologie 25 (1966), 309-315.
(17) U. Moser, I. v Zeppelin and W. Schneider, Simulation of a Model of Neurotic Defence Processes, Beh. Sc. 15 (1970), 194-202.
(18) J. Bastiaans et al., Inst. J. of Psycho-Analysis, 51 (1970), 168-173.
(19) M. Nordström, SLISP - A System for Simulation using LISP, Report DLU 74/35, Dept. of Comp. Sciences, Uppsala University, 1974.
(20) T.S. Brown and R.R. Burton, Multiple Representations of Knowledge for Tutorial Reasoning, in: D.B. Bobrow and A. Collins eds.: Representation and understanding. New York; Academic Press, 1975, 311-349.

Computational Linguistics in Medicine, Schneider/Sagvall Hein, eds.
North-Holland Publishing Company, (1977)

CURRENT TRENDS IN ARTIFICIAL INTELLIGENCE
by

Erik Sandewall
Informatics Laboratory, Linköping University, Linköping, Sweden

The paper makes a short survey of the field of Artificial Intelligence,
combined with the author's opinions about and assessments of develop-
ments in the field. It is intended as background material for the continued discussions at the conference. The style and content of the present paper must be understood in the context of the working conference
at which it is presented. The paper is a combined short survey of the
state of the art in artificial intelligence research, and a position
paper for the interdisciplinary discussions that would take place at
the conference.
As a position paper, it includes the author's assessment of develop-
ments in the field, but the text, the examples, and the references have
been selected for representatives of other fields, rather than for
people who themselves work in artificial intelligence. The reference
list consists mostly of a list of recommended reading in the field.

THE GOALS OF ARTIFICIAL INTELLIGENCE RESEARCH

Many computer based systems today have properties which make them inconvenient
for their final users. These inconvenience-causing properties are often described
and "explained", in general terms, by saying "the computer does not have any intelligence". For example,

- the user must adapt to the system's preferred language of communication,
rather than vice versa

- the system cannot give explanations why it has taken certain actions

- the system cannot handle new and unforeseen situations

Artificial intelligence research is a branch of computer science which attempts
to develop programming technology so that these restrictions can be removed, and
so that forthcoming computer systems become able to communicate more fluently, to
explain their behavior, to handle unforeseen situations, and to exhibit other similar signs of intelligent behavior.

This goal does not per se make it necessary to imitate the "internal design" of
human intelligence, i.e. models borrowed from psychology, in the design of arti-
ficial-intelligence programs. After all, man's first successful flights were made
using balloons, which represent a technique which is entirely different from the
one birds use. However, the experience in AI (artificial intelligence) research
so far has been that antropoid designs, obtained either from the science of psychology or naively through introspection, have turned out to be more successful
than other methods based on e.g. mathematical theory.

One may speculate that the introduction of limited intelligence in computer programs could gradually evolve into artificial systems that display general-purpose
intelligence. This is as serious or unserious as to speculate that today's space
programs will gradually evolve into the colonization of the universe by mankind,
an idea which is not a priori impossible, but which is so remote that it cannot
guide serious research today. AI has inspired a fair number of fantasies, but
should not be identified with them.
Like many other words in our language, "intelligence" is not particularly well
defined. In other contexts we are perfectly willing to use it anyway, and the
context of artificial intelligence is no exception. The general, common-sense
meaning of "intelligence" is sufficient for making "artificial intelligence" a

meaningful term. At least so far, a common design philosophy has seemed useful for accomplishing several different aspects of limited intelligence in experimental systems. In practice, the exact limit of the extent of "intelligence" that is attempted in AI research must be defined partly by the range of applicability of this common design philosophy and common body of methods.

RESEARCH PARADIGMS

It follows from the above that AI is an engineering discipline. It is not the empirical study of existing, "artificially intelligent" systems, but rather the development of a technology.

During the twenty years that the field has existed, several research approaches have been tried. Some may be characterized by the terms "top-down" and "bottom-up", which are widely used in computer science.

The top-down approach to AI would be to start with the abstract goal formulation: "intelligence in computer based systems", and attempt to break it down into sub-problems. One might for example hypothesize that in order to exhibit certain intelligence, a system would have to contain certain program modules and certain data bodies, and then recursively break them down. The bottom-up approach would be to start with some very elementary algorithms and methods which are likely to be useful as components in the final system, study their properties, and build upwards.

Both the pure top-down approach and the pure bottom-up approach have given relatively little reward. The top-down approach tends to result in mere speculation, while the results obtained using a bottom-up approach, although in themselves correct, have quickly been invalidated as irrelevant to the goal. (The largest body of bottom-up work has been done in the study of automatic deduction using resolution).

The dominating methodology is instead to implement limited-purpose systems, in order to develop general methods and principles, and also in order to develop software tools. This interplay is illustrated in figure 1. Research so far has resulted in a common body of general methods and a philosophy for how to do things. It has also resulted in a number of programming systems, auxiliary programs, and other software tools. Each subsequent research project draws on this background in order to implement an experimental system for some chosen application, and develop one or a few aspects of intelligent behavior in that application. If the application is well chosen and the project is successful, it contributes to the general background by adding more methods or tools, or by giving additional experience with existing methods and tools.

Still other paradigms have been proposed, such as simulated evolution, but no significant results seem to have been obtained in that way.

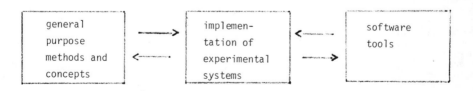

Figure 1

EXAMPLES OF GENERAL METHODS AND OF LIMITED-PURPOSE SYSTEMS

The following table lists a number of general methods which have been developed
in AI research, and some application areas where the methods have evolved. The
crosses indicate the applicability. Thus some application areas draw on several
methods, and vice versa.

	question-answering systems	comprehension of continuous natural-language texts	understanding/debug electronic equipment	mobile robot	mass spectrography	prove mathematical theorems
practical, low-key parsing of natural language	x	x				
assimilation of natural language into a data base	x	x				
representation of natural-language-based knowledge in a data base	x	x		x		
deductive search	x					x
search in a problem space			x	x	x	
scene analysis				x		
pattern matching and fitting of structured data to a given patterns		x	x			

The labels for the methods and the application areas are hopefully self-explanatory. The reference list at the end of the paper gives additional material about
these items. Ref. (1) is an excellent introduction.

TOOLS

The tools mentioned in the third box in figure 1 include:

-    the programming language LISP, and related languages that have been developed
     from it. LISP can be characterized in several ways:

=   it is an interactive, incremental language. In this respect it is similar to APL
=   it is a programmable data-base system which (unlike conventional systems) uses just one logical memory level. The programmer may assume
  that the entire data base is in primary memory, although in practice
  one usually uses paging
=   it is a programming system where the program is stored in the system's
  data base. This makes it easy to write program-analyzing or program-ge-
  nerating programs, and to integrate a program with its associated data
  (such as the data it used, or the data that serves to document the program)
=   it is a programming language for operating on data structures in an
  interactive environment, which means for example that convenient input/
  output of data structures must be defined.

Ref. (1), (2), (3), (4) are textbooks for LISP. Ref. (5) is a survey of LISP programming.

-    programming techniques that are useful in a LISP-like programming environment, such as:

=   techniques for program generating programs
=   flexible data base organization
=   use of auxiliary languages in the implementation of a large system
=   interactive program development techniques

Ref. (5) gives a survey of such programming techniques.

-    very high level languages, which have been experimentally implemented in
  LISP, such as PLANNER, QLISP, and others. Ref. (6) gives a survey of this
  family of very high level languages.
-    auxiliary programs or programming languages based on the frame (7) philosophy, for example KRL ("Knowledge Representation Language") (8)
-    grammar systems which can be viewed as specialized programming languages for
  writing natural language parsing programs, for example the ATNP (Augmented
  Transitional Network Parser) system (9).

RESULTS

An evaluation of the results of research in this field could focus on either of
the three boxes in figure 1. One could either evaluate the methods that have been
developed, or the performance of the experimental systems, or the quality of the
tools. An evaluation of the experimental systems is the most straight-forward
among these.

In doing such an evaluation, one must however keep in mind that experimental systems are developed in order to gain new knowledge about the methods and tools,
and only rarely in order to serve a practical purpose. They are subject to a
principle of diminishing returns: at the point where most of the potential new
knowledge has been squeezed from the experiment, the system would still need a
large amount of additional programming work before it could be put to practical
use. One is usually confident that such remaining work is not difficult in principle, but since it has little research interest it is simply not done. Therefore,
when the performance or experimental systems are used as a measure of progress in
the field, they must be seen as indications of feasible performance, rather than
as completed achievements.

A comparison of experimental systems that have appeared since 1960 show a very
clear and steady rate of progress. Like in many other fields, systems which were
returned as Ph.D. theses in 1963 or even 1968 are fairly simple exercises today,

and current systems are clearly more advanced by several orders of magnitude. Several different reasons have contributed to this progress:

- Better methods. For example, ten years ago each research project in natural language understanding had to develop its own "semantic network" representation. Today one can use an established one.

- Better tools, for example the ATNP systems (9).

- Better understanding for how to use methods and tools. There is a lot of experience, in completed projects, to guide the early top-down design work for each new experimental application.

- Better computer systems, in terms of both reliability, capacity, accessibility, and price. In particular, the possibility to implement and run large programs in LISP has been of decisive importance for many recent projects.

- Greater confidence, There have been a number of projects that set out to build a large, integrated system for doing certain tasks, and which succeeded. That makes it easier to make another attempt and to choose tasks with the right level of difficulty.

NATURAL LANGUAGE ANALYSIS

For the present conference, it is natural to give some particular attention to the work on natural language analysis that has been done within artificial intelligence.

From an engineering standpoint, it has been natural to subdivide the problem of natural language analysis top-down-wise into three successive steps:

- a parsing step which determines the structure of the incoming sentence

- an assimilation step which relates each incoming sentence (or phrase) to the data base of the recipient system. Assimilation includes for example the determination of referents for anaphora, and determining whether a sentence in a narrative text refers to a new event or gives additional information about a previously mentioned event

- an action step which performs an appropriate operation, for example obeys an instruction or answers a question.

It is natural that one should look to linguistics for help in the design of the parsing step, and perhaps also the assimilation step, and to psychology and/or philosophy for help in the design of the data base and the operations on it. Unfortunately there are almost no examples of systems which have been able to use results from psychology or philosophy for this purpose. In the case of linguistics the relationship is more complex. It has changed over time in a fashion which can be appropriately described by the Hegelian paradigm of thesis - antithesis - synthesis.

The parsing step must perform a morphological analysis (determine the root and the ending(s) of each word) as well as a syntactic analysis (determine the parts of speech in a sentence). Especially in the analysis of English language, one has generally assumed that the syntactic analysis was the major problem.

Transformational grammar (originated by Chomsky, (10)) seemed to offer precise models of syntax that could serve as a basis for a parsing program. The intended purpose of that research is to give an insightful explanation of what are the sentences of a language and what are not, where the "insight" requirement has a consequence that the grammar must assign a structure to each sentence.

The question of what is a sentence "in" the language is not altogether clear. For example, should
     "The bachelor wrote a letter to his wife"

be considered as a sentence "in" the language, given that a bachelor is an un-
married man? One possible, generous reaction might be that since it is intuitive-
ly obvious what the parts of speech are in this sentence, it would not hurt to
accept it as being "in" the language. However, this viewpoint has the disadvan-
tage, from the linguistic point of view, that the resulting grammar is also too
generous in its assignment of multiple, false parses to undoubtedly correct sentences. It therefore seemed natural, still from the linguistic viewpoint, to make
the grammar more and more elaborate, in order to pin down more and more narrowly
what are the allowable sentences.
There was of course also another reason for the increased sophistication of
grammars, namely attempts to account for more and more complex sentences.

When researchers in artificial intelligence first considered using these results
from linguistics for the parsing component in their experimental systems, they
usually discarded them for the following combination of reasons:

-     some of the tasks that are taken on by transformational grammars, in order
      to pin down the "correct" language as narrowly as possible, and in order to
      reduce structural ambiguity, can be performed by other parts of the enginee-
      red system. In other words, if the grammar is viewed as a candidate parser
      module, it is overgrown and tries to do too many things. A more even-handed
      division of responsibility between the modules seemed more effective.
      This argument assumed that there could be flow of control and information
      back and forth between the parser and the other parts of the system. A
      "closed" parser, which generates all possible structure assignments and then
      quits, would be unpractical. But modern programming technology allows one to
      write parsers so that they communicate continuously with other parts of the
      system, and thereby can be restricted to generate only one or a few parses.

-     relatively little was known about how to organize the other parts of the
      system, and therefore the entire system could only accept a sequence of
      quite simple sentences. It would then be overkill to use a parser that could
      accept very sophisticated sentences.

-     Nobody had any good ideas about how to implement a parser based on a trans-
      formational grammar with anywhere near reasonable efficiency.

AI research therefore developed an antithetical approach, namely to use simple,
low-key parsers that were tailored to the requirements of the experimental system
at hand. The ATNP system (9) has gained widespread use, and has effectively
enabled everybody to write his own, simple grammar. In some cases, the antithesis
was brought forward as extremist, programmatical positions to the effect that syntax need not be used at all, or only as a last resort when semantic features did
not provide the required information (11), (12).
It seems that we are just now experiencing the synthesis, where AI systems are
starting to feel the need for more ambitious parsers, that can accept a wider
range of sentences, and where linguistics tends to give grammars which are simpler, which are easier to implement as parsers, and which then leave more for
other parts of the total system.

APPLICATIONS IN MEDICINE

Artificial intelligence research may yield applications in medicine both directly,
through systems which are useful in medical practice and which have intelligent
features, and through spin-off effects, where the software tools which have been
developed in AI research can be used for the design of systems which do not have
intelligent features but which have other attractive properties. The MYCIN system
presented at the present conference is the obvious example of the direct application; the LIM system (LISP IMS Manager) which supports the use of an IMS data
base system (13) is an example of a spin-off application.

REFERENCES

(1) Patrick H. Winston: Artificial Intelligence. Addison-Wesley Publishing Co.,
     1977.
(2) Clark Weissman: LISP 1.5 Primer. Dickenson Publishing Col., Belmont, Calif.,
     1967.
(3) Anders Haraldson: LISP Details. Uppsala University (Sweden), Datalogilabora-
     toriet, 1975.
(4) John McCarthy et al.: LISP 1.5 Primer. MIT Press, 1962.
(5) Erik Sandewall: Programming in an Interactive Environment: the LISP Experien-
     ce. Linköping University, Informatics Laboratory, 1977.
(6) Daniel Bobrow and Bertram Raphael: New Programming Languages for Artificial
     Intelligence Research. Stanford Research Institute, 1973.
(7) Marvid Minsky: A Framework for Representing Knowledge, in Patrick H. Winston
     (ed.) The Psychology of Computer Vision. McGraw-Hill Book Company, New York,
     1975.
(8) D.G. Bobrow, T. Winograd: An overview of KRL, a knowledge representation
     language, Xerox Palo Alto Research Center Report, May 1976.
(9) William A. Woods: Transition Network Grammars for Natural Language Analysis.
     Comm. ACM Vol. 13, No. 10, October 1974.
(10) Noam Chomsky: Syntactic Structures. Mouton & Co., The Hague and Paris, 1957.
(11) Roger C. Schank et al.: Margie: Memory, Analysis, Response Generation, and
     Inference on English. Proceedings Third International Joint Conference on
     Artificial Intelligence, Stanford Research Institute, 1973.
(12) Yorick Wilks: Understanding Without Proofs. Ibid.
(13) M. Jainz and T. Risch (eds.): A Data Manager for the Health Information
     System Berlin, Comp. Progr. Biomed. 6 (1976), 166-170.

Computational Linguistics in Medicine, Schneider/Sagvall Hein, eds.
North-Holland Publishing Company, (1977)

SEMANTIC NETWORKS
AND NATURAL LANGUAGE UNDERSTANDING[*]

Carl Wilhelm Welin
Department of Linguistics
University of Stockholm
Stockholm, Sweden

The general principles of semantic networks are
outlined, as well as their use in a natural language
understanding system. The method of partitioning
networks in order to represent opaque contexts and
alternative views of the world is described, and it
is discussed how such elements of the text as quantifiers, intensional predicates, modal auxiliaries,
etc. should be used as signals for initiating and
guiding the network building and scanning semantic
procedures of the language understanding system.
Finally it is suggested that network partitioning
could be used to represent the hierarchical textual
structure of a narrative or an argumentation.

1. Semantic networks

Suppose that we have a store of information about a set of entities
which is organized in the following way. Each entity has a unique
name which serves to identify it. A set of possible binary relations
between the entities is given. There is an information retrieving
procedure which, given the name of an entity and the name of a relation as arguments, will return the names of those entities, if any,
which bear the given relation to the given entity.

New information can be added to this data base if there is another
procedure which, given the names of two entities and the relation(s)
between them, will store this information in a way that makes it
accessible to the retrieving procedure.

If the human eye and brain provide the information retrieving procedure this kind of data structure may be implemented as a network
diagram on, say, a piece of paper. Thus, Figure 1 is a store of
information about the kinship relations between a set of persons.
The nodes of the network represent the entities about which we have
information, and the labeled arcs, or pointers, between the nodes
represent instances of binary relations between the entities. In this
case, a pencil may be used for adding new information to the data
base. If we were using the programming language LISP for implementing
the data structure, the LISP functions GET and PUT would be the procedures for retrieving and adding information, respectively.

When used for storing information extracted from natural language
texts or speech, such relational data bases are often called semantic
networks (Simmons 1973, Hendrix 1975). The reason for using the term

*)This work was supported by the Swedish Humanistic Research Council.

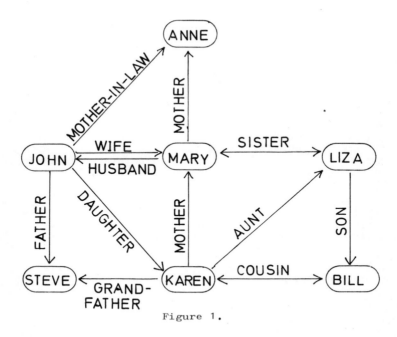

Figure 1.

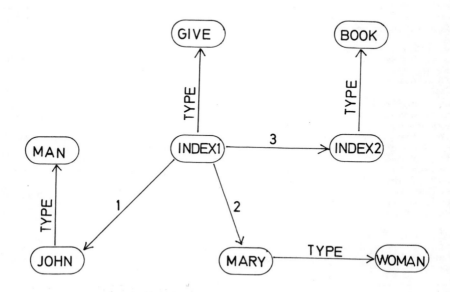

Figure 2.

semantic is not quite clear, but sometimes concepts borrowed from the area of linguistic semantics are used for network relations. In Simmons´ text understanding system the names of deep structure cases (cf. Fillmore 1968) are part of the set of possible labels of network pointers.

There is no generally accepted format for semantic networks, nor is there any sharp borderline between semantic networks and other kinds of information structures that use indexing by means of labeled pointers between data units, such as the Knowledge Representation Language of Bobrow and Winograd (1977). As is suggested by the example above, a semantic network may be implemented physically in many different ways. The essential characteristic is that the information which has been stored, i.e. the set of instances of binary relations represented by pointers between nodes, at the same time provides an indexing of the data base. This indexing makes it possible to scan the network in an associative manner, following the labeled pointers until one finds a node, or configuration of nodes, that represents a relevant piece of information. Clearly, semantic network is a functional notion, i.e. what really counts is how the information retrieving and information storing procedures operate on the network.

2. Natural language understanding

How is a semantic network used in the process of understanding a natural language text? An important part of this process is to establish data units, i.e. network nodes for each one of the entities referred to in the text.

When a new entity is introduced, a new node is created, and pointers are added to represent the relations between that entity and those which have already been actualized by the discourse. These relations may either be explicitly mentioned in the text, e.g. by means of prepositions, or implicit and intended by the author to be understood as the 'normal' relationships between such objects. When an old entity is referred to once more, it is identified with an already existing network node by its description in the text. This description very often mentions known relations to other entities, so it is seen that the associative method for scanning the network along the pointers for the correct node corresponds fairly well to the way natural language is used when referring.

Lexical and grammatical features of the text are used as signals for initiating and guiding the network building and network scanning procedures of the language understanding system. For instance, an indefinite noun phrase in the text generally signals that a new entity is being introduced, while a definite one signals that the node of an already mentioned entity should be looked for in the network, or alternatively, that the referent of the noun phrase is implied by the context or well-known to anyone.

Implied by the context means that objects of this kind normally occur together with something that has been explicitly mentioned in the text. In the following example the church is implied as soon as the village has been mentioned, and so on.

(1) Last Saturday we went to a village nearby. The church was closed, but the vicar opened so we could admire the paintings.

It follows that the semantic analysis procedures should have access to generic information on entities that normally belong together and the nature of their relationship. Whether this information should be

organized as a set of individual inference rules, as so-called frames
(Charniak 1975), or in some other way is still an open question. It
should be noted, however, that the simplistic type of semantic network we have been discussing so far is not able to store specific and
generic information side by side.

The reason why we establish nodes corresponding to the referents of
the noun phrases of a sentence is that these nodes are the places
where the information given in the sentence about those referents
should be stored. This is the purpose of the nodes and pointers
device, namely that all information about any one entity should be
readily accessible from its node, and still one should not have to
duplicate any piece of information in the data base.

Until now we have been assuming that all kinds of information about
entities can be represented as labeled pointers between network
nodes. However, if a sentence contains a predicate having more than
two arguments, such as give in

(2) John gives Mary a book,

it is of course impossible to represent the predication as a binary
pointer between two nodes. One will have to use a separate node for
the predication and pointers from this node to the nodes representing
the arguments. The same solution, a predication node, is necessary if
an instance of a relation occurs as an argument of another predication, as in

(3) John knows that Paul loves Mary,

or if one wants to represent e.g. the fact that an event occurs at a
certain time.

Since there may be more than one instance of giving, knowing, loving,
etc., and also more than one book in the universe of discourse, the
corresponding natural language words cannot be used as names of
nodes. For this purpose unique identifiers are generated, such as
INDEX1, INDEX2, INDEX3, etc. They correspond to the referential in-
dices of theoretical linguistics. Moreover, to show what kinds of
entities the nodes represent, pointers labeled TYPE, or perhaps
ELEMENT, will point to other nodes the names of which will be GIVE,
KNOW, LOVE, BOOK, etc., as in the network representation of sentence
(2) in Figure 2. It is not quite clear what kind of entities these
latter nodes represent, whether it should be the set of all events of
giving, etc. (Hendrix 1975), the psychological concept of giving, or
some other entity with still more dubious ontological status.

Similar problems will be met with when we try to represent instances
of one-place predicates. To represent the referent of the noun phrase
a red book it will be necessary either to introduce a node for the
concept of redness in general or the set of all red entities, or else
to abandon the semantic network principle that all information about
entities should be representable as binary relation pointers between
nodes. So it seems that the notion of semantic network becomes much
less clear when one tries to apply it to natural language understanding. Certain properties of phenomena can only be described as binary
relations to other entities in a rather farfetched manner.

3. Network partitioning

As mentioned above, we probably have to introduce network nodes representing a general concept, or the set of all entities having a
given property. However, except for these concept nodes all nodes of

an ordinary semantic network have in a sense the same status as regards the reality of the objects they represent. Unless certain nodes
are flagged in some way or other, the information retrieving procedures will not be able to distinguish nodes of hypothetical entities,
such as the referent of a unicorn in

(4) John believes he saw a unicorn in the garden,

or nodes corresponding to existentially quantified variables within
the scope of a universally quantified one, such as the node of
a book in

(5) Every student borrowed a book,

from the nodes of real or specific entities, such as e.g. John.

For information retrieval purposes it is necessary to distinguish
nodes having different ontological status. Another reason is that the
difference in status is reflected in the grammatical structure of the
text, as we shall see later on.

One of the most interesting attempts to solve this representational
problem is Hendrix´ (1975) proposal that semantic networks should be
partitioned into network spaces, or hierarchically embedded subnetworks. These subnets are collections of nodes representing all kinds
of entities, as well as of relation pointers between the nodes. There
is no limit to the possible depth of embedding, and several subnets
may be embedded inside a common superordinate one. In Figure 3 subnet
S3 is embedded in S2, which is embedded in S1, and so on. Each subnetwork is associated with a uniquely named node in the next higher
network of the hierarchical structure.

The 'outlook' of the language understanding system can be located inside any subnet. In an actual implementation a certain global variable of the system will then point to the node associated with that
subnet. That the whole of the semantic network is viewed, say, from
inside subnet S3 in Figure 3 means that new nodes which are created
by the system will belong to this subnet, and also that the information retrieving procedures will only find information that belongs
to S3, S2, or S1. Information of subordinate or coordinate networks
will not be seen, nor will facts of superordinate networks that are
explicitly contradicted in S3. This kind of hierarchical data structure can also be created in CONNIVER, QLISP, and similar high level
programming languages.

When a subnet is used for representing a hypothetical world created
with such a predicate as believe, want, dream, etc. the predication
node will have an argument pointer pointing to the node associated
with the subnet. All nodes inside the subnet represent phenomena belonging to, say, the belief world of the subject of the predicate,
and the pointers represent supposed relations between these phenomena
as well as to phenomena outside the belief world. Cf. Figure 4, which
is a sketchy representation of example (4).

When the subnet is used to represent a universally quantified or conditional statement, the nodes of the subnet will be construed as existentially quantified variables within the scope of the universally
quantified variable. The subnetwork may be regarded as a kind of
'mini-frame' (cf. Charniak 1975), which can be instantiated when
something is found which matches the universally quantified variable
– this would be the way to make an inference by means of a general
rule stored in the semantic network.

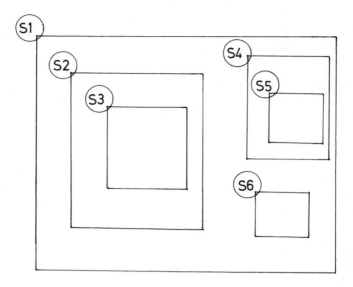

Figure 3.

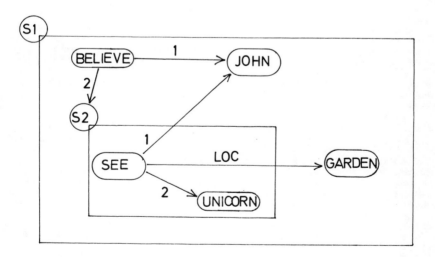

Figure 4.

Hendrix also seems to suggest that network partitioning may be used to encode time relations (1975, p. 3). Bearing in mind the outlook device described above, it is clear that a series of subnetworks, each of them embedded in the preceding one, could represent the successive states of a situation that changes in the course of time.

4. Building partitioned network structures

In Hendrix´ paper nothing is said about the procedures for creating the appropriate subnets during the parsing of a text, and for changing the outlook of the system from one subnet to another according as the outlook of the text changes. To construct such procedures is of course a very difficult linguistic problem.

As already mentioned in section 2 above, definiteness of noun phrases can be used as a signal for guiding the referential procedures. In the same way intensional predicates, quantifiers, subjunctions, and modal adverbs and auxiliaries may serve as signals controlling the semantic procedures which create subnetworks and change the outlook when needed. For instance, as soon as the quantifier every was met with in a text, as in

(5) Every student borrowed a book,

a new subnet would be created, and all new nodes would be located there until the outlook was moved out of that subnet. Thus, the node corresponding to a book would end up inside the subnet representing the scope of the quantifier every in (5), whereas in

(6) A student borrowed every book

the node of a student would be outside the scope, i.e. the subnet, of the quantifier, since every had not been found yet when the subject noun phrase was being analyzed by the parser.

(7) There is a TV set in every home.

Unfortunately, the linguistic facts are more complicated than that. In the preferred interpretation of (7), the existentially quantified variable corresponding to a TV set is within the scope of the univer-sal quantifier, although the word order seems to indicate the oppo-site. It is obvious, then, that the whole of a sentence has to be analyzed (in its context, moreover) before it can be decided what subnet structure the sentence should give rise to. It is not possible to have a direct coupling between certain structure building semantic procedures of the language understanding system and the corresponding lexemes, phrases, and grammatical constructions, i.e. a simplistic kind of procedural semantics.

With the same reservations as above, one can use such predicates as want, believe, dream, etc. as network creating signals. As is well-known (cf. Karttunen 1969), indefinite noun phrases in the comple-ments of these predicates are generally ambiguous as regards their referential status. For instance, the noun phrase a Norwegian in

(8) Liza wants to marry a Norwegian

may refer either to a specific Norwegian whom Liza has chosen for her future husband, or to any Norwegian. In such a case two alternative semantic networks have to be created, one in which the node represen-ting the Norwegian is located outside the subnet representing Liza´s wishes (the specific interpretation), and another network structure in which the node is inside that subnet (the non-specific interpreta-tion). When sentence (8) occurs in a text it may be continued in various ways, and normally the continuation resolves the ambiguity:

(9) He should be a banker.
(10) He is a banker.
(11) But she hasn´t found one yet.

One of the functions of the modal auxiliary <u>should</u> is to signal that
an intensional description, such as the one <u>in</u> (8), is being continued. Consequently, if the next sentence is (9) then the outlook is
still inside Liza´s wish world, as opposed to (10) where the plain
indicative shows that the outlook has changed to the real, or rather
the speaker´s world. If (8) is followed by (10), the Norwegian has to
be interpreted as a specific one, and the node representing him has
to be outside the subnet of the wish world. Otherwise it would not be
possible to refer to him with the pronoun <u>he</u> once the outlook had
changed to a superordinate subnet. If (11) follows (8), the combined
uses of the word <u>but</u>, the indicative mood, and the pronoun <u>one</u> signal
that the Norwegian was a non-specific one, that the outlook has now
changed to the superordinate network, and that the speaker is using
this utterance to comment on Liza´s wishes and the actual state of
the world. It is clear that the semantic procedures which build subnets and change the outlook of the system have to take a great many
grammatical **factors** into account, as well as purely pragmatic ones.

Sentence (11) by the way presents a difficulty to the partitioned
network treatment of opaque contexts. Why is it still possible to
refer to the (non-specific) Norwegian with <u>one</u> in (11), even after we
have left the subnet in which the node representing him is located?
It seems that this node is still accessible as a kind of intensional
description, although the information retrieving procedures should
not be able to see it from outside its subnetwork.

In order to solve these problems one may have to introduce an intermediate semantic representation, perhaps similar to the formulas of
intensional logic, which is saved temporarily along with the semantic
network representation during the parsing of a text.

5. <u>Network partitioning and text structure</u>

It should also be possible to use network partitioning to represent
certain features of the supersentential structuring of a coherent
text. As we have seen, a subnet of a semantic network may be the description of a hypothetical situation that is the object of someone´s
wishes, or what would come about if certain conditions were satisfied
and so on. In this manner information from several consecutive sentences is subsumed into a higher level unit and represented on that
level by the node associated with the subnet.

The higher level unit is related to the rest of the content of the
text as an argument of a predication, or the consequent part of a
conditional, etc. In this way the description becomes an element of
another description on the higher level. But the exposition of a text
may be hierarchically structured even though it is not dealing with
hypothetical situations or alternative views of the world.

An obvious example is the practice of dividing the text into chapters
and sections, which are provided with headlines stating their general
content. Another example is a question followed by a sequence of sentences that together make up the answer. In these cases the hierarchical structure is explicitly marked by typographical features and the
grammatical form of the text. But quite often one has to rely on non-
linguistic information to find out what structure the author of the
text intends.

Loetscher (1973) has made an attempt to classify the possible pragmatic relations between a sequence of sentences constituting a description D and a preceding or following assertive sentence S which
functionally is on a level with the description sequence as a whole.
Some of the most common types seem to be the following. S can be a
summary of the general content of D. More specifically, S can be the
speaker's evaluative comment on the content of D, as in Loetscher's
example

(12) The Millers are strange people. Jack has red hair. Bill suffers
     from a nervous tic.

On the other hand it is possible to view the description, i.e. the
last two sentences of (12), as an illustration, an explication, or
even a kind of proof of the first sentence. In texts which have the
purpose of teaching or arguing, the alternations between a statement
of a theoretical principle and a description serving as a proof or
explication of that principle play a very important part.

Several other types may be stated, but these are enough to show that
there is a need for a representational device which makes it possible
to treat information from several sentences as a unit in order to
relate it as a whole to the content of another sentence - or a similar unit - on a higher level.

It seems natural to use subnetworks for this purpose. The nodes contained in such subnets will of course not have the same hypothetical
status as, say, the nodes of subnets representing someone's beliefs.
The status of the referents corresponding to the nodes will generally
be indicated by the manner in which the subnet is related to the rest
of the network, i.e. as an instance of a general principle, or as an
argument of an intensional predicate, etc.

Adverbs, conjunctions, and above all the order of the sentences in
the text are the principal grammatical aids to find out how the exposition of a text is structured. But the overt signals are in most
cases not enough to determine the structure unambiguously. An important part will therefore be played by generic knowledge about possible instances of general principles, what may be regarded as an explanation, and so on. Quite probably one will also need information
about the speaker's opinions and beliefs about the world.

To represent the structure of a narrative or an argumentation is to
store information about some of the intentions of the speaker or
author when making his exposition, and that is of course an important
aspect of language comprehension. But this structuring of the network
may also pose problems to the information retrieving procedures.
Nodes of 'real' entities, as well as hypothetical ones, will be difficult to find if one does not know what roles those entities play in
the argument of the author.

On the other hand, partitioning may be an advantage if persons, objects, and events can be described in brief outline on a higher network level, and the detailed description be stored away in a subnet.
Then the information retrieving procedures could be designed to scan
the network in a superficial manner at first, and then focus their
attention on some particular entity by entering the associated
subnetwork.

References

Bobrow, D.G. & T.Winograd (1977): An Overview of KRL, a Knowledge
    Representation Language. To appear in <u>Cognitive Science</u>, Vol. 1,
    No. 1.
Charniak, E. (1975): Organization and inference in a frame-like
    system of common sense knowledge. Working paper No. 14, Istituto
    per gli studi semantici e cognitivi, Castagnola, Switzerland.
Fillmore, C.J. (1968): The case for case. In E.Bach & R.T.Harms
    (eds.): <u>Universals in linguistic theory</u>. Holt, Rinehart & Winston,
    New York.
Hendrix, G.G. (1975): Expanding the utility of semantic networks
    through partitioning. Technical Note 105, Artificial Intelligence
    Group, Stanford Research Institute, Menlo Park, Cal.
Karttunen, L. (1969): Discourse referents. International Conference
    on Computational Linguistics, Preprint No. 70. Skriptor, Stockholm
Loetscher, A. (1973): On the role of nonrestrictive relative clauses
    in discourse. In C.Corum, T.C.Smith-Stark & A.Weiser (eds.):
    <u>Papers from the ninth regional meeting</u>. Chicago Linguistic
    Society, Chicago.
Simmons, R.F. (1973): Semantic networks: Their computation and use
    for understanding English sentences. In R.C.Schank & K.M.Colby
    (eds.): <u>Computer models of thought and language</u>. W.H.Freeman and
    Company, San Francisco.

Computational Linguistics in Medicine, Schneider/Sågvall Hein, eds.
North-Holland Publishing Company, (1977)

ON THE REPRESENTATION OF NON-PROCEDURAL KNOWLEDGE

Uwe Hein
University of Düsseldorf and Uppsala University Data Center

ABSTRACT

The paper discusses some criteria which should guide the design of a medium for the representation of knowledge. It will be claimed that understanding natural language is not only one process of mapping a given language input into a semantic representation.

Understanding must be regarded as an activity in which a lot of different processes are involved. Therefore, the controlling of the processes and their communication is of the utmost importance.

Within this framework the demands on a medium for the representation of knowledge can be investigated. One of the hypotheses states that there are no principal differences between the representation of facts and events of the external world and the representation of the system's 'mental' domain.

The paper will give a short survey of a three level model for representing knowledge and will then concentrate on expressions for the representation of non-procedural knowledge.

INTRODUCTION[$)]

The main problem involved in designing a medium for the representation of knowledge is to provide flexible structures which can be altered efficiently in the course of processing. This is important, because understandning natural language text is not simply one process of translating the given input into an internal semantic representation. Many processes are involved in that task. They transform the given input almost continuously, assembling it into the system's knowledge base. Even there processing may continue on a later occasion.

The scheduling of the processes involved must be controlled by an operative system which can provide rich control structures. Ideally, the operating system allows a multiprocessing environment where resource allocation, prioriting, and resuming of processes is possible. x)

From this point of view the representation of knowledge has not only to deal with the facts and events of the external world, but must also cover the systems 'mental' domain. It is reasonable to believe that knowledge about the world and knowledge which the system maintains about itself is not principally different.

This perspective on the organization of knowledge has another advantage too. In the construction of understander systems one does not want to work with big and undifferentiated programs. As much of the system's code as possible should reside on clearly defined information structures to be processed by few and general programs. This in only possible if, as stated at the beginning, the structures in question allow the necessary flexibility and generality.

For the following it will be useful to distinguish clearly between the general

---

$) Most of the ideas presented in this paper derive from research done in connection with my doctoral thesis (Hein /3/).
I would like to thank Rolf Pfeifer and Anna-Lena Sågvall for a discussion of this paper.
x) More refinements can be found in Bobrow and Winograd /2/ and Bobrow and Raphael /1/.

principles concerning the form of the representation of knowledge, or the representational medium, and the analysis of certain domains of knowledge. The principles state what kinds of elements can be used and what types of combinations
are allowed. The analysis of a concrete domain of knowledge, on the other hand,
uses these elements and rules to build up cognitive maps of the domain in question.

I shall consider some criteria which should guide the design of a medium for the
representation of knowledge. In order to illustrate these ideas I shall introduce
kappa-expressions which are used for the representation of non-procedural knowledge.

STRATIFICATION OF THE REPRESENTIONAL MEDIUM

Most of the effort at designing the representational medium will be devoted to
the definition of new datatypes which are suitable for a given purpose. Naturally,
these datatypes have to be constructed out of a fixed set of types provided by
the programming system in which the medium is to be embedded. Furthermore, there
may be several steps between the primitives of a programming language and the
highest elements of the representational medium.

In order to come to a clear understanding of what entities are used, which relations exist between them, and what impact one has on another, it is necessary to
start the definition of the representational medium at the lowest level, the
programming language. The next higher level then contains those elements which
directly have been constructed out of the elements of the programming language.
This stratum may even contain entities which have been taken over from the lower
level by simply renaming them.

Renaming certain datatypes may be desirable if one wants to describe the elements
of the higher levels in terms indepdent of the programming system's terminology.
This may be a first step towards clarification and unification of the conceptual
tools.

The process of constructing new layers continues until one reaches the elements
of the highest level. As a result, the representational medium can be described
as a stratified system, where both the influence of the given programming environment on the design of the representational medium and, vice versa, the needs of
the medium with regard to that environment can be traced.

A THREE LEVEL MODEL

While the representation of the last section was quite abstract, I shall give
some illustrations here by presenting the outline of a system for representing
knowledge where three strata are distinguished.

The system is implemented in Lisp, so that the elements of the lowest level are
the datatypes available in Lisp. These elements are called molecules.

```
COGNITIVE UNITS:
        Individuals, Events, Concepts, Facts
----------------------------------------------------------------
COGNEMES:
        Attributes, Kappas, Lambdas, References
----------------------------------------------------------------
MOLECULES:
        Atoms, Lists, Integers, Arrays, Strings ...
```

Figure 1: A stratified description

At the next higher level we find references, attributes, kappa- and lambda-expressions. The elements of this level are called cognemes. References are pointers to cognitive units or other elements of the cogneme level. With the help of attributes properties of a cognitive unit can be described locally.

Lambda-expressions are used for the representation of procedural knowledge. An expression can only be regarded as a lambda if it is directly executable by the system. Kappa-expressions, on the other hand, are used for representing non-procedural knowledge. Later on, I shall consider kappa-expressions in more detail.

Cognitive units form the elements of the highest level. They tie together elements of the cogneme level providing the most stable structures in which knowledge can be expressed. Consequently, the cognitive units have a great impact on the structuring of the momory space. At this level we find concepts and representations of individuals, events, and facts.

KAPPA-EXPRESSIONS

Kappa-expressions are those structures in which most of the non-procedural knowledge is expressed. They are composed out of a category-concept and a set of branches connected with it. Each branch, in turn, consists of binding-concept and a dependent value. The dependent value may be a reference or another kappa-expression. It should be obvious that there cannot exist any limitations to the complexity of the kappa-expressions.

Fig. 2 shows (in a first approximation) two kappas expressing the ideas that peter eats a frog and that the frog is big. The category-concept of the first kappa-expression is ACTION. To the knowledge which is associated with this concept belongs that ACTION is a propositional theme, that it needs at least an ACTOR and a PLAN branch in order to be meaningful, and all the knowledge which can be stated in terms of action, object, actor, and plan (eg. that it is the ACTOR who does something to the OBJECT). Looking at the dominant category-concept in a kappa-expression gives already some information what the whole expression may be about without looking into it.

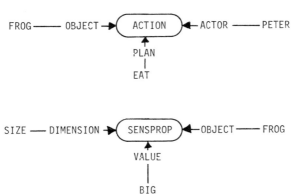

Figure 2:   Two kappa-expressions.

While the kappa-expressions of fig. 2 give a picture of the general structure, they are still incomplete, because the positions of the dependent values are occupied by natural language words (for the sake of simplicity). How the kappa-expressions would really look like depends mainly on the situation in which they would be used. I shall discuss some alternatives which may give an idea about the functioning of the whole.

First of all, Peter is an individual. Either the individual is known and is already located in memory, or it is not yet known, or is not yet identified. In the first case we can use a reference, say I0037, for identifying the individual in question. In the second and third case there must be a description of the individual which contains the given information, but no definite connection to any indivual in the memory. x) Simplified such a description could be represented in form of a kappa-expression:

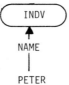

where the category-concept tells us that the kappa-expression denotes an individual.

The same considerations hold for the object of the ACTION-expression, the frog. But here we have one more possible interpretation. 'Frog' could be understood as a concept to allow the generic interpretation. The generic reading (that peter usually eats frogs) would, however, not be represented as an ACTION-kappa. It would, for example, be expressed in a structure whose dominant category-concept was HABIT, or some equivalent concept. 'Eat' on the other hand must be substituted by a reference to its underlying concept, say CO122.

One important aspect of kappa-expressions is that their meaning can be determined by the context in which they occur. The SENSPROP-kappa in fig. 2 with the appropriate values for the bindings denotes a proposition (the frog is big). It may, however, appear as a dependent structure in another kappa-expression, in which case the meaning would be determined by the binding-concept which dominates it. To make things clear let us look what will happen if we insert the SENSPROP-kappa expression in the object position of the ACTION-kappa, as it is shown in fig. 3.

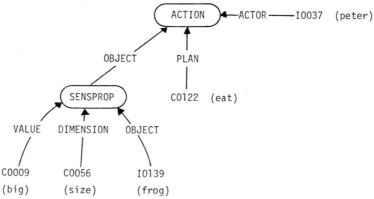

Figure 3:   A composed kappa-expression

x) More generally, every cognitive unit must be describable by a kappa-expression. These descriptions are used for implanting or searching the entities described by the expressions. It is important to stress that the description of a cognitive unit and the unit itself are two completely different entities in the system.

In that case it will be indicated by the binding-concept OBJECT bound to ACTION
that the whole dependent structure designates an object of the action, in which
case the whole expression is to be read as a description of that object. The
meaning of the whole structure could then be paraphrased as 'peter eats the big
frog'.

REQUESTS

In order to show that kappa-expressions are not only used for declarative knowledge as it might be suggested by the examples, I shall demonstrate in this section how questions can be expressed in the same format. I use the term 'request'
to stress that I do not talk about the linguistic entity which is a certain type
of utterance, but about the logical content of a question.

A request might be represented as a kappa-structure whose theme is the category
concept REQUEST. Bindings necessary to make the whole expression meaningful are
TYPE, REQOBJ, and EXP. TYPE specified the type of the request, whether it is a
WH or a YES/NO-request. If it is a WH-request we need a request-object, a certain
entity to search for. EXP binds the underlying proposition. The contents of 'what
did peter eat?' could accordingly be represented as shown in fig. 4. o) For the
same of simplicity I shall use words instead of references within the kappa-expression.

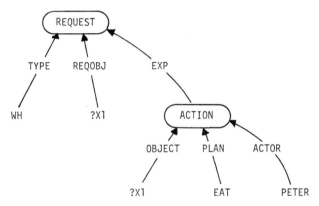

Figure 4:   What did Peter eat?

In searching for an answer the system must take the dependent expression of the
EXP-binding and match it with those expressions that are stored with the individual Peter. The category-concept will be used for a first selection of the possible candidates, the PLAN-EAT branch as a second. The value of a successful match
will finally be bound to the variable X1 which in turn can be used to generate
a response.

FACTS

The last section dealt with kappa-expressions. I want to repeat that kappa-expressions do not express facts, but propositions which represent only one part of the
truth.
A fact is a cognitive unit consisting of a proposition and a set of attributes.

o) Disregarding any time concepts involved.

One, and the most important, is the truth value telling us whether the propositions or its negation fits into the world.

Other attributes are the origin and the consequences. The origin tells us where
the information comes from, from a perception or a conclusion from another fact.
The consequences specify what conclusions have been drawn from this fact. Usually
much more information will be associated with a fact, as with every cognitive unit.

FRAMES?

Nowadays it seems to be quite impossible to write a paper on the representation
of knowledge without mentioning frames. It is, however, my conviction that this
notion, how suggestive it might be, does not give us any new insights into the
nature of semantic relations. Let me, as an example, discuss how concepts contribute to the understanding of a situation and how this knowledge can be modified
by exceptions specified as knowledge about individuals.

Fig. 2 in this paper gives a kappa-expression which is intended to represent an
idea like 'Peter eats the frog'. We have seen that the dependent value of the
PLAN-binding is a reference to the concept EAT. Pointing to the concept EAT means
that all the knowledge that is stored with the concept is also retrievable from
the kappa-expression. The knowledge about the concept EAT is described in facts
that use a lot of generic concepts, like that one usually eats with fork and knife,
placing the food on a plate and much more. In the context of Peter's eating, the
representation in fact tells us that Peter realizes a plan. It is an individual
realization which might have its pecularities.

One must combine the general knowledge centered around the plan with the knowledge
about the person to find out what the whole situation might look like. These pecularities are then described as exceptions to that general knowledge. It is in
fact the dialectic relation between the individuals and the concepts that allow
that knowledge about a certain situation can be used sensitively, where much of
the sources for the knowledge must be assumings and guessings.

CONCLUSION

While kappa-expressions are used for the representation of non-procedural knowledge, lambda-expressions describe the system's procedural knowledge. In many
situations it will be necessary to transform processes in their descriptions and,
vice versa, transform the description of a process into an executable procedure.
This task conforms to the transformation of kappa-expressions into lambdas and
the other way round. An understanding of these transformations will certainly increase the efficiency of every understander system. There is a good hope that
these questions can be solved in the framework presented in this paper.

REFERENCES

/1/ D.G. Bobrow and B. Raphael: New Programming Languages for AI Research,
    SRI, Artificial Intelligence Center, Technical Note 82, 1973.
/2/ D.G. Bobrow and T. Winograd: An Overview of KRL, a Knowledge Representa-
    tion Language, to appear in Cognitive Science, Vol. 1, 1977.
/3/ U. Hein: Semantik und Kognition, Düsseldorf, to appear in 1978.
/4/ D.A Norman and D.E. Rumelhart: Explorations in Cognition, San Fransisco:
    W.H. Freeman and Co., 1975.
/5/ R. Schank: Conceptual Information Processing, Amsterdam: North-Holland, 1975.

Computational Linguistics in Medicine, Schneider/Sågvall Hein, eds.
North-Holland Publishing Company, (1977)

CRITERIA FOR
CLINICAL DECISION MAKING

M N Epstein and E B Kaplan
Section on Medical Information Science
University of California
San Francisco, California

This paper describes a knowledge representation model and a process model for clinical decision making. These models motivate the specification of criteria which may be used to compare medical decision making methodologies. The criteria are grouped by decision process, knowledge representation, and explanatory capability. Some of the issues discussed include goal-directed utility-driven search strategy, hierarchical problem definition, and mapping functions between entities.

INTRODUCTION

A prerequisite to progress in developing systems which will accomplish higher order processing in medicine is the definition of a framework to describe the medical decision making process and associated knowledge representation. Review of the literature on the subject and study of existing systems using artificial intelligence, computational linguistics and statistical methods confirm that the problems are very complex. To answer the question, "What is the current status of our ability to represent knowledge in a computer?", we must first ask what do we need to represent, and how is this knowledge to be used? This leads naturally to a requirement for criteria to define the necessary tasks and goals.

In this paper we define a generalized model of clinical decision making which embodies a knowledge representation model, a patient data base, a process model for manipulating elements in the knowledge representation and data base, and a translation model for interacting with the "outside world". These conceptual models are used to motivate a preliminary set of criteria. The insights derived from these criteria are directed at answering our initial question.

PREREQUISITES FOR CRITERIA DEVELOPMENT

First, it is necessary to provide a general framework within which the clinical decision making process may be viewed. In our subsequent development of the criteria, reference to issues of implementation or whether the indicated tasks are performed by man or machine are ignored.

Figure 1 displays a potential framework composed of four modules: the decision-making module, the input module, the question-answering module, and the data base. The focus of this paper, the decision-making module, can be loosely conceived to model the rather elusive concept called "clinical judgment". This module embodies the processes and knowledge necessary to

35

arrive at clinical decisions.

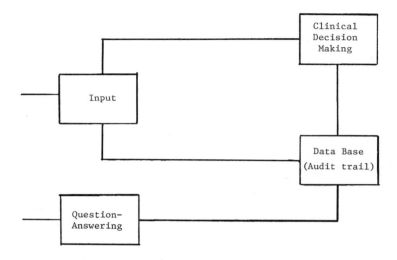

Fig. 1

The function of the input module and the question-answering module is to
interface the decision module with the outside world. The major role of the
input module is to preprocess the data that are to be used in the decision
process. It is expected to handle paraphrases of medical concepts as well as
synonymous concepts. The input module accepts both patient-specific data and
control information which activates or terminates the clinical decision making
process. The question-answering module allows access to the data base about
an individual patient including the intermediate steps by which a decision is
made. The data base contains patient specific data and retains an audit trail
of the context within which each data item is acquired and used.

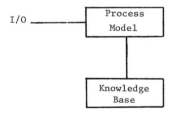

The internal structure of each of the modules, with the exception of the data
base, consists of a process model and a corresponding knowledge base. The
process model performs the basic task of hypothesis selection and
verification, while the knowledge base contains those elements and relations
pertinent to the problem domain. An example of a schematized process model and
knowledge representation for the decision-making module is shown in Figures 2
and 3.

Figure 2 summarizes the clinical decision making process that has been
discussed in various texts by several medical educators such as Walker(1973),

Harvey(1976), and Elstein (1976b). The basic flow consists of successive
iterations through the functional blocks of data acquisition, data analysis,
and plan formulation with associated feedback between functional boxes.

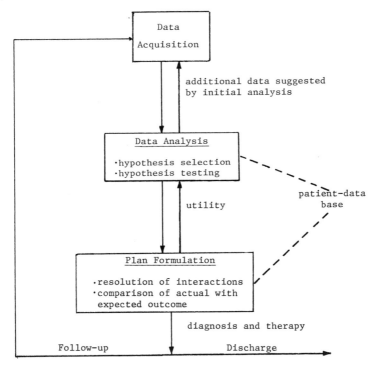

Fig. 2. Process Model – a functional description

The process begins with the collection of a minimal number of data elements
pertinent to the patient's status, data analysis terminates explicitly after
one or more iterations with the realization of the goal of diagnostic or
therapeutic determination, or implicitly without an adequate decision due to
limitations of medical knowledge or available data. The overall process
terminates only when the patient exits from the process in some manner.

The goals of this process are to determine the answers to the following
questions: What hypotheses are being considered?, and what should be done
next? For each problem, the following need to be considered:
1. Should the patient be referred?
2. Is the problem sufficiently defined to allow therapy?
3. Does the severity of the problem require immediate, prompt,
   elective or no therapy?
4. Is therapeutic adjustment required?
5. Is diagnostic reevaluation required?

In addition, for each set of problems it is necessary to determine:

1. Are there therapeutic or diagnostic interactions? and
2. Are they significant enough to require resolution?

Several issues are raised by this process model, and by work that has been conducted in the area of information processing. The most prominent of these is the necessity for reducing the size of the search space both in terms of hypothesis selection and verification. It is noteworthy that studies indicate that physicians consider only four to five hypotheses, and that a hierarchical nesting of hypotheses is used to both drive data collection and increase information storage capacity. (see Elstein (1976a), Wortman & Kleinmuntz) Furthermore, even at this level of generality, several points emerge. First, diagnosis is by no means synonymous with clinical judgment, but only a portion of it. Second, diagnosis is affected heavily by factors other than the probability of the hypotheses being considered. As indicated, in figure 2 the expected value or utility of the outcome plays a significant, perhaps dominant role in directing the diagnostic search. Third, feedback plays a central role in this process, and addresses the inherently non-deterministic nature of clinical medicine. In this setting discrepancies between actual and expected results are used to control diagnostic reevaluation and therapeutic modification. Finally, resolution of interactions (both positive and negative) between diagnostic and therapeutic maneuvers is essential in all but the most trivial of cases.

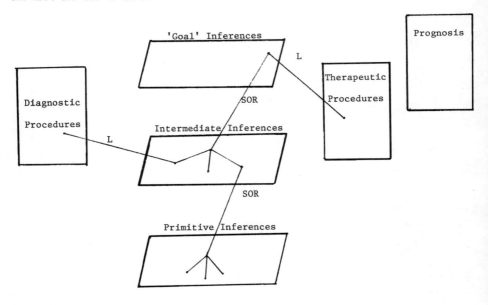

Fig. 3. Knowledge Representation Model
(L = Link   SOR = Strength of Relation)

Figure 3 is a generalized knowledge representation model modified from the work of Kulikowski and Weiss (1976). This model provides a conceptual structure for the knowledge base which is associated with the previously described process model. The function of the knowledge base is to provide a static representation of the entities and the potential relations between entities that can be accessed during instantiation of the process model. This representation can be viewed as levels of abstraction consisting of a set of planes, and mapping functions between and within planes. The planes are ordered hierarchically with the most primitive observations or entities in the lowest plane, intermediate inferences based on observations in the middle plane, and what might be thought of as "terminal" or "goal" inferences in the upper planes. These have been divided into disease states, prognosis, and therapy.

An example from malignant melanoma, an area in which we are currently doing work in natural language question-answering can serve to illustrate these ideas. Suppose we have a patient with a dark mole which was noticed 6 months ago, and has been bleeding intermittently for the past several weeks. The lesion is ulcerated, approximately .5 cm. in diameter and there are no palpable lymph nodes. These represent the primitive inferences. The intermediate inferences might be ulcerated nevus and no lymph node involvement, while the terminal inference might be possible malignant melanoma. This sequence of inferences represents the process of hypothesis selection, and corresponds to moving from higher to lower order inference planes. The decision might be made to gather additional data or to initiate a specific therapy or to wait. The option to be selected will depend on the weight of evidence supporting this hypothesis, as opposed to others, and the possible therapeutic and diagnostic maneuvers available. Requests for additional diagnostic data can be generated by descending from the higher to the lower order inferences that potentially support them. This corresponds to hypothesis verification and provides a natural way of grouping the data to be collected. In this case a punch biopsy might be considered as a diagnostic maneuver, while a wide reexcision might be considered as a therapeutic maneuver. The probability and value of the outcomes associated with various alternatives must be weighed to determine the action to be taken. Note that even in this simple example the interaction of the knowledge base and process model is essential.

As this example illustrates, there is a need to represent relations between and within levels of inference in a flexible manner, as well as estimates of probabilities for outcomes and complications of potential maneuvers.

CRITERIA DEVELOPMENT

The features of the clinical decision making model composed of the input, question-answering, and decision modules, now serve to motivate the development of a list of criteria. These criteria define some of the requirements to accomplish medical decision making. The objective here is not to determine which methods are "good" or "bad" or whether one method is sufficient to accomplish the entire task, but rather to discern the areas in which a given methodology might be profitably employed. Furthermore, some perspective regarding the magnitude of the overall task may emerge.

Figure 4 lists the criteria related to data acquisition, data analysis, and plan formulation modules discussed earlier. An example of each criterion will serve to illustrate its meaning.
    Sequential data aquisition means accepting a single datum at a time in response to a question as "How old are you?" Parallel data acquistion refers to multiple data items being accepted at once as with a physician presenting a

summary of findings on a patient.

Criteria Name	Related Issues
A. DATA ACQUISITION	Sequential and parallel data acquisition
B. DATA ANALYSIS	
1. Goal Directed, Utility Driven	Change in probability and value of outcome with context
2. Hierarchical Definition of Problem	Relationship between levels of disease
3. Self-correcting Hypothesis Selection	Account for unmatched data, missing data, 'red herring' phenomena, error in problem level definition
4. Grouping of Orders	Timeliness of results, follow-up evaluations
5. Diagnosis of Concurrent Diseases	Relationship between diseases (causality, association)
C. PLAN FORMULATION	
1. Recognition of Interactions Between Hypotheses	Resolution of conflicts, optimization of therapeutic and diagnostic maneuvers
2. Modification of Therapy or Diagnosis Based on Outcome	Determination of prognosis and outcome

Fig. 4.   Process Model Criteria

A goal-directed utility-driven search strategy implies that the ultimate goal of treating the patient, rather than complete data collection or diagnosis, directs the search. The decision to obtain further diagnostic information, or treat is driven by the expected value of the outcome of each of these options. This strategy requires knowledge not only of the various outcomes, including side effects and complications and their "probabilities", but also of the values of these outcomes from the patient's point of view. An additional complication is that the utilities (expected values) are also a function of time. For example, the value of a transfusion may be high if administered in the next ten minutes, while it may be valueless if given in one hour.

Hierarchical definition of the problem is coupled closely with the structure of the knowledge representation. Since complete knowledge is rarely available, a given problem may start out as palpitations, and be refined in light of further evidence as cardio-vascular disease, arrhythmia, paroxysmal atrial tachycardia.

Self-correcting hypothesis selection is related to the notion that in areas of imperfect knowledge and data, errors are likely to occur and their effects must be minimized. Atypical presentations of disease, such as bacterial endocarditis with negative blood cultures (absence of a common finding), or the presence of an erroneous finding such as "bloody urine" in a patient who in fact has red urine due to eating beets (a "red herring"), must not irrevocably perturb the hypothesis selection-testing cycle. Furthermore, if the initial data suggest a specific diagnosis, say hepatitis, but later evidence contradicts this, consideration of other more appropriate hypotheses should occur.

Grouping of orders is exemplified by ordering a set of laboratory tests as opposed to sequential single requests. This is important both in terms of time efficiency and in test-reordering for follow-up. For example, evaluation of a suspected cerebral vascular accident may require a neurologic examination, EEG, lumbar puncture, and brain scan.

Diagnosis of concurrent illnesses is often required, and their relationship may be important to management. For example, in a patient presenting with hypertension and renal disease, management would be very different if the hypertension were caused by the renal disease, rather than the two being merely concurrent.

Recogniton of interactions between hypotheses is essential to avoid potentially deleterious results. Giving penicillin for a strep throat to a patient allergic to the drug would be an example.

Modification of diagnosis and therapy based on outcome information is probably the largest task from the point of view of patient care. This criterion implies not only an ability to do prognosis, and hence establish expected therapeutic or outcome goals, but also an ability to formulate follow-up plans, compare actual with expected outcome, and carry out the appropriate actions.

Criteria Name	Related Issues
A. MAPPING FUNCTIONS	
1. Relations	Causality, association, proximity, superset, subset, negation, time
2. Strength of Relations	Probability, measure of belief, weight of evidence
B. ENTITIES	

1. Inferences
  - Primitive Inferences
  - Intermediate Inferences
  - "Goal" Inferences
	Links to procedures, arithmetic relations

2. Procedures (Tests)
 	
  - Diagnostic
  - Therapeutic
	Probability and value of outcomes and complications in context
	a priori reliabilities

Fig. 5. Knowledge Representation Criteria

Figure 5 lists the criteria associated with the knowledge representation model (Figure 3). The criteria are of two types, mapping functions and entities. Several examples will serve to illustrate some of these ideas.

The following is an example of the different types of prototypes: ulcerated skin lesion, malignant melanoma, and malignant melanoma stage II, are primitive, intermediate, and "goal" inferences respectively.

Excisional biopsy and therapeutic lymph node dissection are examples of diagnostic and therapeutic procedures.

Inferences must also be linked to related procedures. For example, malignant melanoma would be linked to excisional biopsy, while malignant melanoma stage II would be linked to lymph node dissection. Arithmetic relations, such as depth of invasion greater than .5mm must also be represented as an entity.

Procedures have associated with them outcomes and complications which have probabilities and values. For instance, lymph node dissection has outcomes of positive or negative nodes as well as the possible complication of infection. The probabilities and values (how worthwhile the outcome or complication is) will change depending on the context in which the procedure is performed.

Diagnostic procedures also have reliabilities associated with their outcomes. That is, when a pathologist reports positive nodes, his judgement may be correct only 95% of the time.

Most of the relations are well known and have been discussed elsewhere (Feinstein (1967), Hayes (1973)). Strength of relations have been treated in various ways from data base determined probabilities, to subjective probabilities, to certainty factors, to measures of belief. All apply some semi-quantitative measure to the relation. For example, high mitotic rate is associated with poor prognosis in 70% of cases. The strength of the relation is 70%.

Several criteria follow from the other modules in figure 1. The question-answering module provides a capability to explain the intermediate steps in the decision making process. The input module implies a language process capability to interface the user with the models. These capabilities can be viewed along a continuum from indexing to sophisticated language comprehension. The work of Pratt described at this workshop are indicative of this approach.

DISCUSSION OF CRITERIA

A set of criteria have been proposed. It is now worthwhile to reflect on their consequences. First, several global issues are considered. Although in the previous section the process and knowledge models were developed independently, it is important to note that in the clinical decision making process there is a dynamic interaction between these models. Another observation concerns the relationships of statistical and AI approaches to the generalized models. While the basic models have as their genesis an artificial intelligence approach, other methods can be viewed in the context of this global framework. For example, in the Bayesian approach, goal inferences and primitive inferences are elements of the knowledge representation. The mapping function between these inferences is Bayes' rule itself which yields a posterior probability or liklihood of a goal entity given the primitive entities.

Several of the criteria noted above, although of importance in the practice of medicine have received limited attention in heuristic approaches proposed to date. These criteria may indicate areas in which further study is desirable. These areas include follow-up and therapy recommendations and implementation of utility-driven decision making methods. A short discussion is now given for each of these items.

The follow-up portion of the plan formulation criterion is very important from a medical standpoint. Without belaboring the point, it may be concluded that the problems of follow-up and therapy have received far less attention compared to diagnosis than is their due, and work in this area may be profitable. An example which apply utilities to therapeutic problems might be treatment of an uncomplicated acute urinary tract infection with an antimicrobial without verifying the nature of the organism. The reason for pursuing this strategy is that the utility of obtaining further diagnostic information is less than that of treating presumptively. This illustrates the idea of a utility-driven goal-directed strategy. Looking beyond the field of AI, we see that this problem has been addressed theoretically in decision analytic research. It is worth emphasizing that while potentially powerful, it is difficult to accurately estimate the large number of required probability and outcome values. Within the domain of AI there is as yet no work which duplicates that of the decision analysis formalism. However, at a recent conference at UCLA on clinical judgment an idea emerged that might be applicable. Essentially, the idea addresses the problem of exceptions to general rules. For instance, "a coin lesion in the lung is a tumor until proven otherwise", where "otherwise" denotes a potential list of rare or less severe exceptions to the rule. Notice that implicit in this statement is an ordering of hypotheses by expected value. That is, even though malignant tumor may not be the most probable, its importance is such that it is searched for first. In this way "reasoning by exception" may be used to modify or change a conclusion or action. This approach may provide a method for heuristic specification of utilities.

In describing the consequences of the knowledge representation criteria, it is worthwhile to briefly consider two representations currently prominent in artificial intelligence systems, that is, productions and variations on the general theme of networks. The work of Shortliffe (1976) uses productions as a representation for fuzzy knowledge. This representation has proved to be powerful and led to impressive performance in consultations for bacteremia.

The network representations used in the work of Kulikowski and Weiss (1976), Pauker et al (1976) and Pople et al (1975) are of importance. The networks used are inference nets, rather than the pure semantic networks that have found application in language understanding. The power of semantic networks and partitioned semantic networks (see Hendrix (1976)) are representations worthy of further study to represent medical knowledge. The work of Duda et al (1976) and Shortliffe and Buchanan (1974) provide useful ways of measuring belief and developing formal methods for modeling uncertainty.

Hierarchical relations are easily represented in a network formalism, but are more difficult to represent as production rules. Statistical techniques have not dealt with nor do they seem capable of handling the superset or subset relation.

The fact that primitive inferences are defined in a somewhat arbitrary manner raises the issue of specifying the reliability of the input data. For example, hepatomegaly meaning an enlarged liver is often considered a primitive inference. However, there are other problems such as emphysema that may also produce a similar finding of palpable liver without being associated with hepatomegaly.

In considering mapping functions, it is significant to note that efficient solutions of complex problems occasionally involves multiple approaches or viewpoints. This suggests that redundant representations with different organizations or multiple paths between entities may be a necessary implementation characteristic. In terms of Figure 3, this can be looked at as skipping levels.

The criterion that has received much attention in the AI literature is the capability of programs to explain their actions. This is especially important in the medical environment where physicians must take responsibility for information generated by machines. In concluding, it is clear that the solution of the overall task of clinical decision making is immense. To gain sufficient depth and new insights into the decision making process, current work has restricted the scope of the problem domain.

CONCLUSION

This paper describes a generalized model of clinical medical decision making which includes a knowledge representation model and process model for manipulating elements in the representation. These models motivate a preliminary set of criteria which define several of the tasks necessary to answer the question "What needs to be represented and how is this knowledge to be processed?" The criteria fall into two major groupings— processes and representations.

Some of the criteria include goal-directed utility-driven search strategy, hierarchical definition of the problem, recognition of interactions between hypotheses, and modification of diagnosis or therapy based on outcome information. Representation of fuzzy or uncertain relations between entities and coupling of entities to their related diagnostic or therapeutic procedures are also discussed.

References

Davis, R. & King, J. (1975) An Overview of Production Systems, Memo AIM-271, Artificial Intelligence Laboratory, Stanford University, 38 pp.
Duda, R.O., Hart, P.E. & Nilsson, N.J. (1976) Subjective Bayesian Methods for Rule-Based Inference Systems, Proc. 1976 National Computer Conference, Vol. 45, 1075-1082.
Elstein, A.S. (1976a) Clinical Judgment: Psychological Research and Medical Practice, Science, Vol. 194, 696-700.
Elstein, A.S. (1976b) An Analysis of Medical Inquiry Processes, Final Report to the Division of Physician Manpower, DHEW, Washington D.C.
Feinstein, A. (1967)   Clinical Judgment, Robert Krieger Publishing Company, New York.
Harvey, A.M. (ed.) (1976) The Principles and Practice of Medicine, Appleton Century Crofts, New York.
Hayes, D.G. (1973) Cognitive Networks and Abstract Terminology, J Clin Computing, Vol. 3, 110-118.
Hendrix, G. (1976) The Representation of Semantic Knowledge, Chapter 5, in Speech Understanding Research, Walker, D. (ed.), Final Report, Stanford Research Institute.
Kulikowski, C.A., Weiss, S., Trighoff, M. & Safir, A. (1976) Clinical Consultation and the Representation of Disease Processes: Some AI Approaches, Rutgers University CBM TR 58.
Pauker, S.G., Gorry, G.A., Kassirer, J.P. & Schwartz, W.B. (1976) Towards the Simulation of Clinical Cognition: Taking a Present Illness by Computer, Amer J of Med, Vol. 60, 981-996.
Pople, H.E., Myers, J.D. & Miller, R.A. DIALOG: A Model of Diagnostic Logic for Internal Medicine, Proc 4th Intnl Joint Conf on AI, 848-855.
Shortliffe, E.H. (1976) Computer-Based Medical Consultations: MYCIN, American Elsevier, New York.
Shortliffe, E.H. & Buchanan, B.G. (1975) A Model of Inexact Reasoning in Medicine, Math Biosc, Vol. 23, 351-379.
Walker, H.K., Hurst, J.W. & Woody, M.F. (eds.) (1973) Applying the Problem-Oriented System, Medcom Press, New York.
Wortman, P.M. & Kleinmuntz, B. Memory and Problem-Solving, Dept. of Psychology, Northwestern University, ms.

Computational Linguistics in Medicine, Schneider/Sågvall Hein, eds.
North-Holland Publishing Company, (1977)

THE USE OF CATEGORIZED NOMENCLATURES
FOR REPRESENTING MEDICAL STATEMENTS

A. W. Pratt
Director, Division of Computer Research and Technology
National Institutes of Health, PHS, DHEW
Bethesda, Maryland 20014, USA

The data found in a medical report or record are almost exclusively of the form
of natural language. These data are supplied by a large, multidisciplinary work
force consisting of a host of professional and paraprofessional medical staff.
As medical circumstances require, each of these workers report the observations
obtained from the conduct of an examination, a procedure or a test in the natural
language terms used to describe the subject matter of the respective medical
specialty involved. Modern medicine comprises many medical specialties each having
its own specialized subject matter vocabulary. The elements of these vocabular-
ies together with the many general language terms required for linguistic expression such as prepositions, articles, modifiers, verbs and so forth, constitute
the vocabulary of the medical language that is common to all natural languages.
The consequence is that the vocabulary of medical language is enormous in size
measured in any human terms. But in spite of this vocabulary problem, a number
of computer-based, medical data processing systems have attempted to provide facilities for the capture, storage and retrieval of natural language medical data
|1-9|. These medical information systems are based on clever strategies involving
computer programming, word processing and content indexing using medical terminologies.

Medicine has traditionally used medical terminologies and truncated medical dictionaries as the basis for representing the content of medical reports, records
and publications. |10-16|. These terminologies form the basis for identifying
and assigning content words and word sets to any document. These content descriptors serve to index the documents for storage and retrieval in an archive. Included among these terminologies are classification systems such as the International Classification of Disease (WHO), categorized nomenclatures such as the
Systematized Nomenclature of Pathology (SNOP), and the word dictionaries and
thesauri used for simple text matching of which the "Lamson Thesaurus" is an
excellent example. The entries in these terminologies serve only as pointers and
therefore, it has been the tradition to exert considerable care in selecting the
terminology entries such that they represent (point to) more global areas of
medical information. Consequently, the entries in the structured terminologies
fail to represent the "fact content" of a document. Word dictionaries and thesauri fail to represent or organize the fact component of a medical document;
they serve largely to identify text which contains target words or target word
sets. The categorized nomenclatures appear to offer the better basis for indexing medical documents while at the same time preserving the summary fact components of the several medical memoranda that constitute a medical record. The
international experience gained from the manual encoding of surgical pathology
reports using the Systematized Nomenclature of Pathology (SNOP) certainly tends
to support this view. The basis for this contention emerges from an examination
of ·the SNOP nomenclature.

The SNOP nomenclature consists of approximately 15,000 specific and medically related pathology terms in English language form. The terms are either individual
words such as "lung" or word phrases such as "lower lobe of the right lung." The
pathology terms include the names of the elemental entities necessary for the
description of pathology such as lung, inflammation, and fibrosis, plus the names
of more global pathology concepts such as "diabetes mellitus," "tetralogy of
Fallot," and "rheumatic heart disease."

The SNOP terms have been divided into four highly structured lists known as Topography, Morphology, Etiology, and Function. It is convenient to define the lists in the following way:

Topography--a list of the names of the body sites. (T-terms)

Morphology--a list of the names of structural changes that occur in tissues as a result of disease. (M-terms)

Etiology   --a list of the names of causative agents of disease such as microorganisms, drugs, and chemicals. (E-terms)

Function   --a list of the names of the physiological manifestations associated with disease plus a limited number of specific infectious diseases. (F-terms)

A SNOP term is assigned to only one of these lists.

The Systematized Nomenclature of Pathology further differs from the other medical terminologies in that it imposes an explicit semantic structure on the domain of discourse that it defines. Each list in the nomenclature represents a categorization of the SNOP terms. The categorization is based on the general usage function of the terms to achieve description of pathology data. Each list is highly structured; related terms are listed together as the semantic content of the terms demands. Each language term in the nomenclature is defined by a five-character code equivalent; the first character designates list membership, and the remaining four characters denote the position of that term in the list. For example, the synonym code for myocardium is T3301. The T marker denotes that MYOCARDIUM is a member of the Topography list or category. The term INFARCT has the synonym code of M5470. The M marker denotes that INFARCT is a member of the Morphology list (category).

By virtue of the categorization of the SNOP entries into the four category lists, the structure of the vocabulary is unambiguously described by a small set of semantic/syntactic elements, namely, "T," "M," "E," "F." These semantic markers indicate the general meaning of any term and, interestingly enough, can provide the same semantic function for equivalent data strings in other natural languages. Quite clearly, the combinatoric use of the T, M, E, F terms affords a rich potential for creating an indefinitely large set of fact-based, subject matter specific medical language statements that can serve well to index a pathology report while largely preserving the fact component of the report. A simple example is sufficient to show the indexing process. Given the language string 'infarct of the myocardium' the SNOP marking process would yield

INFARCT (M5470) of the MYOCARDIUM (T3301)

Similarly, the language string 'staphylococcal abscess of the skin' would be marked

STAPHYLOCOCCAL (E1600) ABSCESS (M4000) of the SKIN (T0100)

The semantic/syntactic markers, T, M, E, and F are absolutely essential to this indexing process or descriptive process. The numeric codes are of limited concern; these synonym markers can be replaced by any systematized scheme of a user's choice. The codes play no role whatsoever in the language processing; the codes do serve well, however, to enhance data processing particularly with respect to file structure and data retrieval.

The SNOP nomenclature representation of pathology data can for data processing purposes be represented as a simple fixed format file structure that incorporates the implicit notion that the nomenclature terms are to be used combinatorically for data description. The file structure would comprise some fixed order of the referenced SNOP terms such as, for example

T-term   M-term   E-term   F-term   = SD

which is called a 'TMEF' statement and is considered to be a semantic description, SD, of the data. The data MYOCARDIUM, INFARCT is represented as

    T3301   M5470   E0000   F0000   Myocardium Infarct

The language string MYOCARDIUM INFARCT is the semantic description, SD, and is stored with the semantic representations of the data.

A patient described as having a CARCINOMA (M8103) of the BRONCHUS (T2600) is represented as

    T2600   M8103   E0000   F0000   Bronchus Carcinoma

A representative record of the pathologist's findings is represented by multiple 'TMEF' statements, viz

T2600	M8103	E0000	F0000	Bronchus, Carcinoma
T0000	M0000	E6927	F0000	Tobacco (Cigarettes)
T0000	M0000	E0000	F7103	Paroxysmal Nocturnal Dyspnea
T5600	M8106	E0000	F0000	Liver, Metastatic Carcinoma
T5600	M3850	E0000	F0000	Liver Hemorrhage
T0000	M7051	E0000	F0000	Cachexia
T0000	M0000	E8816	F0000	Fluorouracil Therapy
○	○	○	○	
○	○	○	○	
○	○	○	○	
Txxxx	Mxxxx	Exxxx	Fxxxx	(Language String)

An extended data retrieval system has been written for use with this SNOP-based archive of pathology data. Data retrieval from a fixed format file structure is a straightforward matter and is a subject that has been treated extensively in the computer science literature thus needs no comment here.

The T M E F statements compose a fixed formatted record which can be readily processed by the computer. Note that, for retrieval purposes, Boolean concatenation of the data can be easily made (1) within a categorical information field, or (2) within the complete T M E F statement, or (3) across several T M E F statements. Perhaps more important is the fact that the T M E F statements reflect the complete categorical domain of the SNOP nomenclature and that the T M E F statement form can provide a complete indexing or coding structure for pathology data limited only by the completeness of the nomenclature. A user of the system is provided with a relatively comprehensive yet simple query language with which to interrogate the data base. A query-request consists of a query-specification section and a query-statement. The query-request allows the user to partition a file and to select those patient-records that fulfill a specified set of conditions. Query-statements range from a simple statement to compound statements using logical connectors. The query language is not a natural language system but consists of structured T M E F statements and the necessary logical connectors. The query language is a "target language" of the natural language encoding system used to recognize and encode the natural language pathology data (discussed below). The presumption is that a query to the system entered in natural language should be analyzed and structured as if the query language represented data to be entered into the file. In this fashion the recognizer/encoding computer programs can act as an on-line editor for "system comprehension" of language style and nomenclature completeness.

The proved adequacy of the SNOP nomenclature for indexing pathology data and the existence of a computer-based facility for retrieval of the SNOP encoded pathology data focused attention on the encoding aspects of the pathology data information system. Manual encoding of these data is a tedious, boring, and costly task subject to a variety of human-induced variations. Automatic encoding would have the very desirable advantages of rapid and consistent encoding of the data and would ensure that the encoding procedures were compatible with the pathology data storage and retrieval portions of the information system.

It was recognized at the outset, however, that developing a "machine intelligence" --that is, a set of computer programs that could satisfactorily mimic the best performance of the human encoder--represented a formidable problem. The pathologists, in common with most medical specialists, use an unrestricted natural language text form to communicate and record pathology data. These text-based messages are usually telegraphic in style in that they are information-rich but word-brief. The competent human encoder can accept and comprehend, for indexing purposes, the meaning contained in the unrestricted natural language text. An acceptable machine-based encoder must perform at a comparable level to be acceptable to the pathologist.

An automatic encoding capability has been developed at the National Institutes of Health (NIH) for surgical pathology data recorded in the unrestricted natural language text form of American English.|17| The computer programs accept and index as T M E F data structures the identical language text used by the pathologist to record his summary diagnostic portion of the medical record. The pathologists judge that the encoder accurately indexes 80 to 85% of the language data. This estimate of competency involves only a very limited number of pathologists from outside the NIH. Thus, there is insufficient evidence for judging the adequacy of the encoder for global use because language usage habits can vary enormously among pathologists. The experience to date does make it obvious, however, that an automatic encoder of high competency can be written from any limited group of pathologists whose language usage habits are known.

The description of the encoder is in terms of coordinated sets of opposed processes. For example, a process facilitating or increasing indexing may be associated with one which reduces imprecise or redundant indexing. Processes described together are not necessarily temporally contiguous in the algorithm.

A brief sequential exposition is as follows on the encoder:

> The encoder breaks a diagnostic statement down into its component words and punctuation which it stores in list form.

> By look-up in auxiliary dictionaries, information is associated with each list item, classifying it syntactically, and controlling subsequent SNOP dictionary look-up for the diagnostic statement.

> Encoding dictionary (SNOP) look-up is performed for the entire diagnostic statement. A dictionary entry is matched when each of its component words can be generated from words of the statement and substitution rules associated with them.

> The codes resulting from SNOP dictionary look-up are combined into TMEF statements which compose the document surrogate.

The basis of the encoder is the assumption that the categorical nature of the SNOP nomenclature affords a competent *semantic model* for indexing pathology data for high precision retrieval. Support for the assumption was gained from the earlier experiment which demonstrated that more than 95% of a large sample of pathology data could be adequately indexed by the T, M, E, or F data elements.

The performance of the encoder relies exclusively on the strategy of recognizing the T, M, E, and F elements in the language data and mapping these elements, according to specific combinatoric rules, to the T M E F data structure of the stored file. The basic encoding process is apparent from the indexing of the straightforward diagnostic statement:

RETICULUM CELL SARCOMA, STOMACH

The key STOMACH is fully matched within the SNOP nomenclature entries:

Stomach Nos*	T6300
Stomach Anterior Wall	T6324
Stomach Greater Curvature	T6322
Stomach Lesser Curvature	T6321
Stomach Lymphatics	T0962
Stomach Posterior Wall	T6325
Stomach Skin Combined Sites	T6390
Stomach Wall Nos	T6323

to yield the index of

Stomach Nos	T6300

Permuting the key phrase RETICULUM CELL SARCOMA is easily done to obtain an exact match within the SNOP nomenclature entries:

Sarcoma Periosteal	M8823
Sarcoma Reticuloendothelial	M9723
Sarcoma Reticulum Cell	M9643
Sarcoma Small Cell	M8803
Sarcoma Spindle Cell	M8803
Sarcoma Stromal Nos	M8933
Sarcoma Synovial	M9043
Sarcoma Undifferentiated	M8803

to yield the index of

Sarcoma Reticulum Cell	M9643

*Nos should be read as "not otherwise specified."

The T and M synonym codes are then listed in the assigned fields in the T M E F data structure:

    T6300   M9643   E0000   F0000   Stomach, Sarcoma Reticulum Cell

and the indexing is completed by listing the E and F fields as null and also listing the SNOP nomenclature English language strings as shown above. The resulting data structure provides an unambiguous semantic statement suitable for machine processing and for the human reader.

An uncomplicated dictionary match of the pathologist's language data to yield a clear indexing statement as in the above example occurs for approximately 25% of the data. The majority of the data require that the encoder perform some degree of syntactical or semantic disambiguation of the language data before a match of the language data against the nominative singular terms and phrases in the SNOP nomenclature can be obtained.

Consider the plural forms of the English language as shown in the following diagnostic statement:

HEMORRHAGES IN LUNGS, OVARIES, AND KIDNEYS

The encoder indexes this statement as

T2810	M3850	E0000	F0000	Lung Right Nos, Hemorrhage Nos
T2850	M3850	E0000	F0000	Lung Left Nos, Hemorrhage Nos
T7102	M3850	E0000	F0000	Kidney Left Nos, Hemorrhage Nos
T7101	M3850	E0000	F0000	Kidney Right Nos, Hemorrhage Nos
T8701	M3850	E0000	F0000	Ovary Right, Hemorrhage Nos
T8702	M3850	E0000	F0000	Ovary Left, Hemorrhage Nos

The encoder properly identifies and records in the data file the right and left members of these paired organs, thus providing the basis for explicit retrieval from the data file. The diagnostic statement

FOCAL INFLAMMATION AND FIBROSIS, CONSISTENT WITH CHRONIC
PYELONEPHRITIS, LEFT KIDNEY

is indexed by the encoder as

T7102	M4302	E0000	F0000	Kidney Left, Pyelonephritis Chronic
T7102	M4805	E0000	F0000	Kidney Left, Fibrosis Focal
T7102	M4800	E0000	F0000	Kidney Left, Inflammation Foxal Nos

and provides an example as to how the encoder develops implicit data for indexing.
Note that both FIBROSIS (M4800) and FOCAL FIBROSIS (M4805) have been indexed. The
adjective FOCAL has been joined with the noun FIBROSIS which follows the conjunction AND. This implicative structure in which an adjective modifies both nouns
joined by a conjunction is a common structure in the English language.

American English has an enormous capacity for paraphrase--that is, the capacity
for rewording or restating a sentence or an utterance without loss or distortion
of meaning. The result is that the same semantic concept can be represented by
different language text having varying syntax. A simple example serves to introduce this complex problem. Note that the following five simple noun phrases:

> Muscle Atrophy
> Muscular Atrophy
> Atrophic Muscle
> Muscle, Atrophy
> Atrophy of Muscle

equally well represent the pathology concept involved. It follows that the indexing of these equivalent data must be identical, irrespective of the differences
in the text strings. It is clear from the example that recognition of the
syntactical keys such as "of" in the phrase

> Atrophy of Muscle

or the comma in the phrase

> Atrophy, Muscle

can provide essential keys for organizing the dictionary look-up and identification of the substantive pathology terms. The more difficult problem is recognizing the adjectival terms which the pathologists are prone to use to create
their brief, information-rich summary diagnostic statements. For example, the
pathologist usually writes STAPHYLOCOCCAL ABSCESS or LARYNGEAL BIOPSY, as opposed
to ABSCESS DUE TO THE STAPHYLOCOCCUS and BIOPSY OF THE LARYNX. Correctly encoding
the semantically equivalent adjective forms such as STAPHYLOCOCCAL and LARYNGEAL
is crucial, since they represent pathology concepts that can be the central data
items of a subsequent retrieval request. Expanding the dictionary to include both
the adjectival and nominal forms of the dictionary entries is, however, an unrea-
sonable solution to the problem. The dictionary would have to grow enormously in
size and would complicate the actual processing of the data with respect to the
on-line storage capacity required and the number of dictionary accesses. Further
it would be an enormous task to prepare manually an exhaustive list of adjectival
forms.

The problem has very largely been solved by the development of an algorithmic mor-
phosemantic transformation strategy which converts the adjectival form to the
nominal form by substituting the adjectival suffix with a nominalizing suffix |5|.
For example, the term LARYNGEAL can be converted to the noun LARYNX by substitut-
ing an "X" for the terminal string -GEAL. Thus, the diagnostic statement

LARYNGEAL BIOPSY POSITIVE FOR EPIDERMOID CARCINOMA

is accurately indexed by the automatic encoder as

T2410   M8703   E0000   F0000   Larynx Nos, Carcinoma, Epidermoid

A tree for the suffix substitution strategies has been prepared and incorporated
into the automatic encoder. The entire tree contains approximately 95 suffix-
algorithm rules and has obviated the need to include many thousands of adjectival
forms in the dictionary; it allows the pathologist the use of unrestricted text
for construction of his diagnostic statements.

Representative of the entire tree is the L-tree portion shown below which lists
the adjectival suffixes recognized by the encoder, which end with the letter "L"
plus the allowable substitutions.

Adjectival		Nominal
L	substituted by	Null
AL		A, E, UM, US
NAL		Null
EAL		US, ES
IAL		US
CAL		X, CUS
RAL		Null
GEAL		X
CEAL		X
ICAL		IX, EX, ERY
ORAL	*	UR
INAL		EN

It will be noted that some of the adjectival suffixes are allowed more than one
substitution with the result that more than one word will be formed in the transformation process. For example, the term CORTICAL will yield by substitution the
term CORTEX plus the *noise* words CORTIX and CORTERY. (See the above list.) Only
the term CORTEX is in the dictionary, and thus the noise words are discarded. All
terms formed by transformation are matched against the dictionary; if the morpho-
semantic transformation yields more than one valid term, the encoding process
ceases and the error is recorded for inspection. Formation of multiple valid
terms is not a problem for the existing tree. It should be clearly understood that
the transformation strategy described above has been carefully devised for mapping
on the SNOP vocabulary exclusively. If the adjectival-to-nominal transformation
strategy is to be used with any other vocabulary, a new set of rules (tree) will
be required to reflect the content and structure of the new vocabulary.

The challenging problem at hand is the capture and explicit recording of the meaning of a pathology diagnostic statement. It is clear that the general language
terms which link the pathology terms in a diagnostic statement contain significant
information with respect to the pathology findings. These terms, which are predominantly prepositions and participles, specify association, cause, effect, negation, and qualification, and are necessary to achieve full disease description.
The experience gained in the automatic encoding of pathology data strongly suggests
that the basic T M E F data structure is adequate for the indexing of the subject
pathology data but requires that this basic data structure be expanded to incorp-
orate the semantic relations which link the T M E F terms in a T M E F statement
as well as links between related T M E F statement.

Formal representation of the extended data structure can be represented in elementary logic. Consider a set, V, of elements called the vocabulary. A binary relation in V is defined as the set, R, of ordered pairs $<x,y>$, where x and y belong
to V. The proposition that x stands in the relation R to y is denoted by xRy.

The SNOP vocabulary consists of the previously defined sets of terms belonging to

the categories T, M, E, or F. Two relations that are useful in pathology diagnostic encoding are L and I. The relation L would have such values as "in" or
"contained in"; the relation I would have such values as "caused by" or "due to."
Using the notion of binary relations, we can write related pairs of categories as

$$m_j L t_i$$

where m_j is the jth term in the set of M-terms;

$\quad t_i$ is the ith term in the set of T-terms; and

$\quad L$ is the relation holding between m_j and t_i.

This data representation can be written as $L(m_j, t_i)$ and would be read as "the jth
lesion in the ith body site." Similarly, the data representation $I(m_j, e_k)$ would
be read as "the jth lesion caused by the kth agent." This concatenation of the
elements of the semantic categories can be expanded to include the entire T M E F
statement to yield a semantic description, SD, of a pathology diagnostic statement. For example, a pathology diagnostic statement which enumerates a body site,
t_i, "containing" a lesion, m_j, "due to" an etiological agent, e_k, "associated with"
a physiological abnormality, f_1, could be represented as

$$A\{I[L(t_i, m_j), e_k, f_1\} = SD$$

The data statement can be rewritten as a primitive semantic network, namely

$$T_1 - 'L_1' - M_1 - 'I_i' - E_1 - 'A_1' - F_1 = SD_1$$

These semantic descriptions, SD_1, can be concatenated to yield higher-level semantic descriptions of the pathology of disease. Presumably, the successive concate-
nations of the semantic descriptions, SD, could be continued to any level of data
representation commensurate with the pathologist's information needs. The computer imposes no limitation on the concatenation process; methods can be developed
to process data which can be cast in terms of the formal data structure shown
above.

Clearly, the limitations on this logical process of creating complex information
structures will relate to the medical content of the data. The pathologist will
have to define, in terms of medical content, the allowable relations among the
semantic categories T, M, E and F, and the allowable relations among the semantic
descriptions SD which describe disease pathology. At the core of the pathologist's
problem of defining medical content lies a linguistic problem. The language tokens
and grammatical forms which represent the defined relations will have to be identified and categorized as to their explicit semantic values. The linguistic con-
ventions used for categorization must be suitable for the cortical perception of
man and the internal representation in the machine.

References

|1| P.A. Shapiro: ACORN--an automated coder of report narrative, Methods Inform.
     Med. 6, 153 (1967).

|2| R.L. Gell and H. Becker: Klartextanalyse pathologischer Biopsiebefunde mit
     Bildschirmabfrage, Methods Inform. Med. 12, 10 (1973).

|3| R.L. Wong and P. Gaynon: An automated routine for diagnostic statements of
     surgical pathology reports, Methods Inform. Med. 10, 168 (1971).

|4| A.W. Pratt and L.B. Thomas: An information processing system for pathology
     data, in "Pathology Annual." Appleton, New York, (1966)

|5| A.W. Pratt and M. Pacak: Identification and transformation of terminal
    morphemes in medical English, Methods Inform. Med. 8, 84 (1969).

|6| B.G. Lamson and B.A. Dimsdale: A natural-language information retrieval
    system, Proc. IEEE 54, 1636 (1966).

|7| H. Jacobs: A natural-language information retrieval system, Methods Inform.
    Med. 7, 8 (1968).

|8| J.C. Smith and J. Melton: Manipulation of autopsy diagnoses by computer
    technique, J.AMA 188, 959 (1964).

|9| A.W. Pratt: Medicine, Computers, and Linguistics, in "Advances in Biomedical
    Engineering" Vol. 3, Academic Press, Inc., New York and London (1973).

|10| Public Health Service: "International Classification of Diseases, Adapted,"
    PHS Publ. No. 1693, Vol. 1, U.S. Gov. Printing Office, Washington, D.C. (1967).

|11| E.T. Thompson and A.D. Hayden, eds.: "Standard Nomenclature of Diseases and
    Operations." McGraw-Hill, New York (1961).

|12| National Institutes of Health: "Medical Subject Headings, Index Medicus,"
    NIH Publ. No. 72-265, Vol. 13, Part 2, National Library of Medicine, U.S. Gov.
    Printing Office, Washington, D.C. (1972).

|13| B.G. Lamson, B.C. Glinski, G.S. Hawthorne, J.C. Soutter, and W.S. Russell:
    Proc. 7th IBM Med. Symp., Poughkeepsie, New York, pp. 411-426, (1965).

|14| R.A. Côté, Chm.: "Systematized Nomenclature of Pathology," Committee on Nomen-
    clature and Classification of Disease, College of American Pathologists,
    Chicago, Ill., (1965).

|15| M. Wolff-Terroine: SABIR-C: automated system of bibliography, information and
    research in cancerology, Bull. Bibliogr. FR 15, 169-176, (1970).

|16| B.L. Gordon, ed.: "Current Medical Information and Terminology." Amer. Med.
    Ass., Chicago, Ill. (1971).

|17| G.S. Dunham, M.G. Pacak and A.W. Pratt: Automatic indexing of pathology data,
    in press, J.Amer.Soc. for Inform.Sci., (1977).

Computational Linguistics in Medicine, Schneider/Sagvall Hein, eds.
North-Holland Publishing Company, (1977)

TERMINOLOGY AND NOMENCLATURES

M. Wolff-Terroine
Department of Scientific Information
Institut Gustave-Roussy
Villejuif (France)

A rapid overview of the problems of medical terminology with
attention on their implications with automatic text processing. The anarchic growth of classifications is showed with
emphasis on the need of compatible structures.

When you question an engineer, a linguist, a geologist on terminological
problems in his field, each of ones will answer that the terminology is specially difficult to treat in his peculiar field. Meanwhile, it seems that the
medical language will be still more imprecise and ambiguous than the others
scientific or technical languages. And this phenomenon accelerated in the
last decades, rendering the problems of terminology more and more difficult to
solve.

During many centuries, the medical vocabulary is growing slowly. Then the
nineteenth century, together apostle of the progress and preserver of the tradition, has forged and admitted new terms, while quibbling about mixed etymo-
logies and linguistic misalliances. The twentieth century, vowed to trepidation
and immediate action does not waste any time for grammatical discussions, it
grasps the word, never mind if it is lame, with blind eye it adopts enthusias-
tically syndroms and theories.

Since thirty years the medicine has been completely overturned. Illness
that was common becomes now rare, the ones that was exceptionnal is now familiar, tropical fever appears in London or Paris. New technics changed the face
of medicine and surgery, medical biology took wing, biochemistry developped
medical chemistry and knowledge and development in nuclear physics are giving
their first fruicts. Radiological investigations bring us audaciously precious
informations ; endocrinology, cardiology, neurology were deeply transformed.
We attend a real explosion of conventionnal medicine : for expressing it, the
physician needs new words. He must indicate the chemical compounds he has to
identify, the plasmatic balance he has noted, the clusters he has caught, the
theories what can explain pathological states, systemic diseases, organic reac-
tions, the hypotheses that justify a treatment ....

During these last thirty years, we attended a great transformation of medicine that accordingly gave rise to an enrichment of medical terminology. We
must go fast, save time, precede the neighbour, create rapidly the word, forge
it, good or bad, but the main thing is that it exists.

I — THE TERMINOLOGY AND ITS PROBLEMS

Then it is interesting to study the medical terms and their etymological genesis and that for three reasons :

- the words carry in themselves the vestiges of earlier civilisations and successive conceptions of medicine and biology and are in that manner a part of our heritage ;

- if we want to process automatically medical terms and to analyse them by algorithms, we must know how they are built ;

- the constitution of nomenclatures and of classifications that could be used by various users and applied to various uses assumes at first a study and an agreement on the meaning of the used words.

This terminological problem has not to be minimized. International bodies, and specially the International Council of organisations in medicine and health (CIOMS) realized its importance for about fifteen years, as an experts group conclusions are showing : "the difficulties of information processing and retrieval are now great barriers to carrying out scientific research. Failing complete synonyms list in the main vehiculary languages in medicine, the information is indexed around the world under different forms with the same meaning so that it is difficult, or even impossible for an user to make it out. The communication in medicine becomes more and more inconsistent because authors and teachers are calling the same concept by various names that are often not well-known for the common reader, or that are incorrect, obsolete of for some other reasons, productor of confusion".

Most diseases are described under several names, some under as many as 20 or 30 different synonyms. The same drug is often listed under numerous different names too. As the tragedy of thalidomide most clearly showed, a drug cannot be rapidly identified unless it has a universally understood and accepted name ; that is, an international non-proprietary name. The same confusion prevails in fields as different as bacteriology, virology and medical chemistry and nearly in all the medical sciences. Sometimes, misunderstandings arise not as a result of any disagreement in principle but simply for semantic reasons. This situation is likely to last for a long time, making general agreement and further progress well nigh impossible and hampering the retrieval of information.

What are the principal reasons of the actual difficulties ?

We could find four main factors

- the specialisation :

At the beginning of 20th century, all the terms of the medical vocabulary were practically understanble for all the doctors. Now the hyperspecialisation has completely changed the situation : the language of a radiotherapist is not understood by a psychiatrist and reciprocally. And even inside the same speciality identical terms have not the same acceptations.

- the multidisciplinarity

In order to set up his diagnosis, to realise his therapeutic indications the doctor must use a lot of disciplines that are not his own : genetics, immunology, biochemistry, and he will use very specific terms without knowing always the real and underlying meaning of these terms.

> - the role of the different <u>schools</u> of <u>medical thought</u> in front of the inherent <u>lack of precision</u> of many <u>medical concepts</u>

We have seen in the last thirty years an internationalisation of medicine : the meetings abound, exchanges of ideas are increased. But we could establish that we are far away from an international agreement for the definitions of medical entities. Words as common as "pathology", "peptic ulcer", "schizophrenia", "botryoid sarcoma" call for different diseases in English, German and French. In the case of epilepsy, the differences of interpretation of the "petit mal" are so large that some specialists attribute to the "petit mal" 3 % of all the forms of epilepsy, when others attribute it 80 % !

We can feel here that terminology is only revealing a problem connected with the essential being of medicine : the difficulty of a consensus on an entity that by itself is not so clearly defined as a chemical compound or a physical phenomenon.

> - the speed of actual evolution of medicine

This swiftness has led to create neologisms sometimes inadequate and quickly out of date. Eponymic diseases and syndroms were multiplied : there are three Osler's diseases, two Recklinghausen's diseases .....! More, the non English-speaking countries have used very often bad translations or adaptations of English medical terms.

The result of all these factors is : a vocabulary with tremendous dimensions of about 200.000 terms, and for definition of which a general agreement is very far to exist.

Then we can see that the medical terminology is plethoric, unprecise and that the meaning of various terms are overlapping : so we can imagine how the direct processing of the words of natural language is difficult for a computer.

The origin and the structure of medical terms

It is commonly said that considering their sources and their modalities of consturction it is easy to break up the medical terms. Is this rule general enough so that an algorithmic treatment could be processed ?

The origins of medical terms are :

- greek-roman terms

   a) as they were or lightly modified

   b) deeply transformed by their transit across Europa

   c) became romans : with greek-latin root but created in Italy, in Spain or in France.

- arab terms

- English terms : they represent a modern contribution which is very important.

Theoretically, from each basic concept the formation of words conserved the purity of language by combining Greek prefix and suffix with a Greek root and likewise for the Latin. In fact many medical terms belong to the both languages. For instance :

Teleradiography is formed with :

Tele	:	at distance	:	Greek
Radius	:	beam	:	Latin
Graphein	:	to write	:	Greek

Though it may also be asked whether the suffix which is added to a basic medical term has always the same meaning.

As said earlier the construction of words has joined significative suffixes and prefixes to term of various origin. So :

- – tomy, – ectomy, – ostomy, – plasty, indicate different surgical technics.

- – itis, indicates inflammation

- – osis, an abnormal condition or a non–inflammatory disease

- – emia, the presence of an element in blood

- a – , the absence of ....

We could multiply examples of such constructions. Yet if we examine in details the terms composed in such a way, we find numerous exceptions : in "hypnosis", what is the value of the suffix "osis", is "thalassemia" really the presence of sea in blood ? In "anuria" the Greek privative "a" has its full meaning, but "anemia" is not the absence of blood, nor "hemophilia", a tropism, an affinity for blood !

It is evident that these decomposition rules as all the linguistic rules have many exceptions. Consequently, if it is wanted, at the occasion of automatic analysis of text, to decompose some words, it is better to refer to a decomposition dictionnary manually done and introduced in the computer.

II – NOMENCLATURES AND CLASSIFICATIONS

The necessity of ordering knowledges and consequently terms which represent them, appeared recently in biological sciences. It is only from LINNE that conceptions began to move in the sense of a classification. However during a long time these efforts were limited to some microfields. The first realisation with a general aim was the International Classification of Diseases. This list of diseases, traumatisms, causes of death, regrouped by etiology and anatomical localisation is destined to the establishment of mortality and morbidity statistics at an international level. This list is not, like many people often believe, a nomenclature of diseases and traumatisms, but a classification done essentially for the statisticians. Moreover it was established in 1855 by the International Congress of Statistics in Paris and is the object of revisions every ten years under the care of W.H.O. It is published officially in English, French, Spanish and Russian by W.H.O.

Much more recently, to remedy to the insufficiency and ambiguity of the usual medical language, classifications and nomenclatures were multiplied in the same time that the use of magnetic support for information storage and retrieval spread out.

Nomenclatures are created for three essential uses :

- bibliographic data banks

- factual data banks (drugs, teaching ...)

- medical record (or parts of medical record)

Several classifications have a large diffusion, such Systematized Nomenclature in Pathology (SNOP), the Index for Roentgen Diagnoses or the Medical Subject Headings of the National Library of Medicine. On the other hand, other classifications don't go beyond the limits of a country, an hospital, or even an hospital department. It shows the particularism of such classifications. An objective data as anatomy is classified very differently in some large classifications of international use !

At the present time we attend an anarchic multiplication of classifications which disagree on :

- the terminology

- the mode of classification of terms (hierarchical structure)

- the mode of representation of terms

So these conditions are giving rise to complex problems when we attempt to organise some works in international cooperation on the basis of medical data. For instance, the Commission of European Communities which is creating a drugs data bank through the coordination of seven existing data bases, is confronted with a very difficult problem of equivalences between the different nomenclatures and classifications which are used.

Actually, in spite of the efforts of bodies as C.I.O.M.S., these difficulties are not going to decrease.

It is normal that classifications and nomenclatures reflect the specific point of view or the specific field they have to describe, but till some limits, and the structure of these classifications could have to autorise an easy conversion from a system in an other.

If we don't keep to some rules of compatibility, the actual situation, which is exactly the same as in Babel tower, will certainly aggravate.

III – <u>NEW TRENDS</u>

   Nevertheless the nomenclatures represent a progress against the anarchy we denounced earlier. But they are not an universeal panacea.

   They have essentially 3 defects :

      1) They require a lot of time for being established. Consequently
         they are expensive.

      2) Their structure are too rigid, reflecting one point of view and
         not the various aspects under which it is possible to consider a
         word. The reality is much more complex and multidimensional.

      3) As consequence of the first two points the nomenclatures and clas-
         sifications are too static and don't reflect the dynamics of
         science : when a classification is a kind of monument, one hesi-
         tates to modify it. Then the updating is difficult and rare and
         always late with regard to evolution of ideas.

   How would be it possible to solve some of these problems ?

   First, it can be conceived to build nomenclatures not manually but automatically. It is perfectly possible now to extract from a set of texts all the
discriminating characters, all the significative words of the concerned discipline. If you submit texts in natural language to a morphological analysis and
after that to some statistical analysis, you will obtain an ordered list with
all the significative terms. This list <u>is</u> a terminology. Many authors have
tried to explore this way, every one proposing a new statistical function.

   At this time what is the best statistics for doing that ? It can be answered : it does not exist. It depends of the conditions of the work : we studied
systematically all the parameters which influence the results, specially :

      – the length of the text

      – the informative density of text

      – the more or less homogeneous character of the concerned text.

   According to the value of these parameters the best statistical technics
have to be chosen. So <u>it can be obtained automatically a terminology.</u>

   But we can go more far. It is also possible to detect in the list you
obtained, the <u>synonyms</u> : if you study the <u>environment</u> of the words you can
calculate all the words in strong correlation with a term. If two words have
the same environment, there is a very high probability that these two words
are synonyms.

   In correlation you can also detect if a word has <u>many meanings</u> : if in
the environment of a word, you discover words depending of different semantic
families, you can affirm that this word has not only one meaning.

For instance, when we consider the environment of the word "precipitation" :

precipitation :
(coagulation   (cloud
(precipitate   (fog
(sedimentation   (humidity
(solubility   (rain
(separation   (snow
                   (rainfall
                   (hydrologic cycle

We can immediately discover that the correlated terms are depending from two different semantic families and that accordingly "precipitation" has two different meanings.

It is also possible to give a structure to this automatic terminology, using some clustering technics. The non-hierarchical methods are giving specially interesting results.

In such a way, it can be seen that it is possible to obtain by algorithms a nomenclature and so to solve the problems we evocated.

But a question can be asked : do we need always nomenclatures ?

We are not sure that they are necessary in all the situations. Of course we need an agreement on the meaning of the used terms. But it can also be conceived that the user will define the semantic relations which are of interest of him. These semantic relations (which are the structure of the nomenclatures), this semantic network, can also be showed by the computer at the moment of the request : all the words with a significative correlation with the initial words of the request can appear on the screen and the user will modify by himself the formulation of the question. With this feed-back method, with two or three iterations, the performances of the data base are largely optimized.

It can be seen that the trends for a next future are very far from conventionnal nomenclatures.

For short and mean term, the nomenclatures will continue to be developped and we have to render them more flexible and to establish some switching device between them.

But for a long perspective, we have the feeling that conventionnal nomenclatures are condemned and that we will develop other methods for representing the semantic network of each medical terms.

PART II

MEDICAL PROJECTS AND APPLICATIONS

Computational Linguistics in Medicine, Schneider/Sagvall Hein, eds.
North-Holland Publishing Company, (1977)

THE HUMAN INTERFACE IN
NATURAL LANGUAGE RETRIEVAL*
Ruby S. Okubo and Baldwin G. Lamson

Introduction

Although digital computers have been in existence for a
quarter of a century, their application in information retrieval
is of recent origin. Most large computer-based information
retrieval systems in the United States date back about ·fifteen
years. A definite trend toward the design of on-line systems,
and conversion of batch, off-line processing to the on-line mode
has been developing since 1970. Users, who have become increasingly knowledgeable, are attracted to the distinct advantages of
rapid response, interactive review, and screening which are
available in on-line search systems.

Although some of the problems of misinterpretation and mis-
communication of batch processing can be avoided, the on-line
mode does not solve all the problems of the batch off-line system.
The user of on-line retrieval systems will face still greater
problems if he is not familiar with the on-line system vocabulary,
the data entry policies and procedures, and the capabilities of
the on-line system's search programs. Unless these problems are
resolved, the quality of user retrievals can be adversely affected
by moving from the batch to the on-line mode.

The interactive session between the medical record analyst
and the retrieval system user, i.e., the human interface in the
UCLA batch Natural Language Retrieval system is analyzed in this
paper in order to identify those factors that would affect the
operation of the present batch retrieval system in an on-line mode.
These factors can then be included in the design of the conversion
to an on-line mode. Interest in artificial intelligence has
directed attention to this possibility of programming the activities of the medical information analyst (Miss Okubo), who has
served as the retrieval system user interface for the UCLA
Natural Language System for the past ten years.

Present Status of Offline System

In April 1977, the Surgical Pathology/Bone Marrow data base
of 179,226 reports contained 2,700,949 words; the Autopsy Pathology data base of 8,661 reports contained 715,243 words; the
Nuclear Medicine data base of 38,950 reports contained 699,543
words, and the Neuroradiology data base of 7,952 reports contained
136,650 words. The total number of reports in all the Natural
Language data bases was 234,794 documents containing 4,252,385
words.

---

*From the Department of Data Processing, UCLA Hospital, Los
Angeles, California

On April 21, 1977 the dictionary contained 17,639 descriptors.
Counts by data base files are as follows:

	Total Frequency	Total Descriptors Used	Words Exclusive to Specialty
Surg. Pathology (incl. Bone Marrows)	2,700,949	11,866	4,873
Autopsy	715,243	9,633	3,022
Nuclear Medicine	699,543	5,251	1,144
Neuroradiology	136,650	3,071	334

The UCLA Pathology Thesaurus of July 31, 1976 contained
15,433 descriptors, 9,393 synonym classes, 5,557 subordinate
linkages, and 229 logical relation terms. The UCLA Nuclear
Medicine Thesaurus of March 5, 1976 contained 4,761 descriptors,
2,803 synonym classes, 806 subordinate linkages, and one logical
relation.

Retrievals have increased from 381 per year in 1974 to 444
in 1975 and 495 in 1976. Since the end of 1975, however, each
routine multiple data base match performed with each update which
counts as one search is made in four copies and is used by Natural
Language users as a source of quality control information.

Increasing demands on the system and major advances in
computer technology made it imperative for us to analyze the
programmable aspects of the human interface in natural language
retrieval.

Interactive Sessions Between the Medical Record Analyst and
Retrieval System User

The purpose of this session is to obtain optimal search
results by eliminating any possibility of false negatives and
minimizing false positives, while keeping computer time and
computer operator handling of retrievals at a minimum, but as a
secondary consideration. During the user-analyst interactive
phase of the search process, no set pattern of questions is
followed. Each answer to a question triggers another spontaneous
reply or question.

The interactive session is conducted as a conversation, not
an interrogation, with some injection of humor or comment about
something that is known about the disease under study. The
purpose is to assist the physician or other retrieval system user
not to tell him what to do, although the net result may be that the
requester asks for some assistance in formulating the free form
narrative request before writing it on the Retrieval System request
form.

Purpose of the Search

Several clues as to what to ask the requester come from
glancing over the search request form. For example, the reason
for the search can indicate whether an exhaustive, fully expanded

retrieval in which all the synonyms and subcategories of the
search terms are referenced automatically from the search system
thesaurus for research purposes, or a limited search for a few
cases to be used as examples of a disease process for a case
conference is needed. If a search has been performed recently
for another requester for the same diagnosis or procedure, a copy
of that search may suffice, and no search need be submitted.
However, if a current updated list of cases is preferred, the
user gets his wish. New users of the system are informed of all
the alternatives available to them, and the system is made to
work for them in every way possible.

Concepts More Important Than Key Words

When reviewing the keyword descriptors listed by the search
requestor, the analyst tries to envision the concept those descriptors represent. In haste, the search requestor may sometimes
select the wrong descriptors; choose general terms when he may
mean to be more specific; or vice versa; or because he does not
know the capabilities of the system, overlook the opportunity to
add frills to the search that will save the requestor's time.

An analyst who is a novice to the system might accept the
request from the user without question and input the search
descriptors exactly as given; or select the wrong key words from
the free form request. Inability to think in concepts and to
relate medical reality with the computer system capability has
been the biggest cause of search failures in the natural language
system. Technical considerations such as, misspellings; inatten-
tion to detailed instructions, inability to group descriptors
logically, and improper placement of parentheses between search
descriptors have caused additional problems with search results
in the past.

Our experience has shown that even with careful monitoring
of an inexperienced analyst the badly formulated searches produce
a false positive rate of 9.6 percent and a false negative rate of
0.1 percent. This performance is not considered catastrophic,
but can be improved. Our 1976 false positive rate for all files
and all kinds of "good searches" is 2.6 percent with no false
negatives (Table I). Inclusion of results of the fifty-four "bad
searches" raises the overall false positive rate to 3.37 percent.

Specificity

A quick perusal of the free text request form often indicates
what the search expression should be. Since a descriptor like
TUMOR is a concept which can be expanded from the Thesaurus to
include 600 synonyms and subcategorical terms, an attempt is made
to determine whether the physician needs a breakdown into benign
or malignant tumors, or even further within one of those categories
to a specific kind of benign or malignant tumor. Thus, when
faced with highly general terms, the search analyst typically
asks a series of questions designed to determine the requestor's
real need for a level of specificity.

TABLE 1
NATURAL LANGUAGE SEARCH STATISTICS

Calendar Year 1976

Files and Kinds of Searches	Total Searches	Total Cases Retrieved	Number of False Positives	% of False Positives	Number of Searches with False Positives	% of Searches with False Positives
Routine Searches						
Surgical Pathology	300	54,954	1,534	2.79	136	45.33
Autopsy	104	7,358	148	2.08	26	25.00
Nuclear Medicine	10	3,473	72	2.07	1	10.00
Neuroradiology	16	1,301	26	2.00	6	37.50
Total Routine Searches	430	67,086	1,780	2.65	169	39.30
Special Searches						
Simple Crossfiles	10	118	0	0	0	0
Routine Cross-File Match & Summary	29	2,703	0	0	0	0
Associated Diagnosis	4	79	2	2.50	1	25.00
with Match & Summary	17	629	51	8.10	11	64.71
Cross File Match & Summary	5	870	1	0.11	1	20.00
Total Special Searches	65	4,399	54	2.25	13	20.00
TOTAL	495	71,485	1,834	2.56%	182	36.77%

The questioning may also lead from specific to generic concepts: If the request were for ADENOCARCINOMA of the BREAST, the
requestor would be asked whether he wants CARCINOMA of the BREAST,
so that INFILTRATING DUCTAL CARCINOMAS would not be excluded. If
the requestor wishes to study all malignancies of that organ,
then the more generic MALIGNANT TUMORS of the BREAST should be
the final choice of descriptors.

The same interactive process may be used to determine the
site(s) of the disease process; for example, whether INTESTINE
refers to either or both LARGE INTESTINE and SMALL INTESTINE. Or
when the request is for EYE whether the physician wishes to
retrieve involvement of the EYELID and ORBIT as well.

Some requestors say they want everything above, around or
near the specified site. The user's intent is clarified by
asking about prefixes which transform the meaning of the site
descriptor such as SUPRA-, INFRA-, RETRO-, etc. An example of
the necessity for avoiding general conclusions based upon the
needs of prior searches but to treat every request individually
is evident from use of the site descriptor PERITONEUM. One
requester will not want RETROPERITONEUM, while another would want
the PERITONEUM search to include this area.

Another common question is whether or not lymph nodes, blood
vessels, or nerves to the site should be included. Care should
be taken so as not to cause false negatives by excluding these
additional descriptors. As a precautionary measure, another
search may be made to verify that no false negatives occurred as
a result of these exclusions.

Frequency of Occurrence of Disease (or Procedure)

The frequency count of a descriptor within the data base may
be an indicator of the frequency of occurrence of a disease or
condition within the file. This will not be so, in cases where a
disease can be described by a combination of several descriptors.
For example, SCLERODERMA is also described as a multiple word
descriptor, PROGRESSIVE SYSTEMIC SCLEROSIS.

Knowledge about the incidence of a disease within the data
base can prompt the search analyst to ask whether a less restrictive search should be made. For example, the request for IDIO-
PATHIC SUBAORTIC STENOSIS may be input as just SUBAORTIC STEN-
OSIS. Because of the possibility that the data base may contain
site-specific descriptors without directly naming the site, a
request for PNEUMOCYSTIS CARINII PNEUMONIA will be coded PNEUMOCYS-
TIS, or OAT CELL CARCINOMA of LUNG may be recalled by requesting
all records containing the single word OAT.

Different Ways that a Diagnosis or Other Descriptors Can be Described

While the thesaurus of the UCLA Natural Language Retrieval
System will upon request, include many of these possibilities,
the thesaurus linkages are only constructed to designate relationships that are always correct throughout the data base of the

system. To do otherwise, would result in an increase of false
positive results. In individual searches, synonyms or subordinates
are sometimes required that are not included within the thesaurus.
Occasionally, these search formulation inquiries reveal the need
for, and feasability of, additional linkages.

Together, the requestor and the search analyst must try to
think of all the different ways that a diagnosis can be described.
In some instances, reference books are checked to validate combinations of descriptors. If an unusual combination of descriptors
is requested, such discussion clarifies and/or further refines
the search request. If relationships that are not included
within the Thesaurus are required, these are added to the search
request.

If an eponymic syndrome or procedure is the search descriptor,
it is expanded into its descriptive terms. For example, TURNER'S
SYNDROME is expanded to include the terms APLASTIC, AGENESIS of
OVARY, and GONADAL DYSGENESIS.

Or if a request is made for a generic disease entity like
REGIONAL ENTERITIS, the conversation may lead to the inclusion of
descriptors like CROHN's, TERMINAL ILEITIS, JEJUNITIS, OR ENTERO-
COLITIS. The requestor may then ask if the search would include
REGIONAL DUODENITIS or JEJUNOILEITIS. and perhaps he may want to
look at all SMALL BOWEL RESECTIONS as well, some time in the
future. Another user, in addition to these synonyms for REGIONAL
ENTERITIS, may add the diagnosis GRANULOMATOUS COLITIS to the
request.

The thesaurus has proved to be a powerful tool, especially
the synonym and subordinate files. The current Logical Relations
file works well for combinations of descriptors that are not
deeply nested. For example, ILEITIS has the logical relation
INFLAMMATION & ILEUM. When ILEITIS is used as a search term, it
will retrieve diagnostic statements that contain the term ILEITIS
and those that contain both ILEUM (or any one of its synonyms or
subordinates) and INFLAMMATION (or any one of its synonyms or
subordinates).

The logical relations capability, however, has three major defi-
ciencies which are currently being studied for correction: (1)
the logical operator NOT cannot be used in a logical relation;
(2) the automatic inclusion of the synonyms and subordinates of
descriptor in a logical relation cannot be suppressed, as they
can be in a search statement; and (3) logical relations cannot be
nested, that is, a logical relation descriptor is not expanded to
include its own logical relation, if it has one.

A Descriptor Having More Than One Meaning

When a descriptor has different meanings depending on context
or a word preceding or following it, the requestor is asked which
meaning he is expecting to retrieve from the data base. For
example, does his request for CYSTECTOMY mean BLADDER EXCISION or
EXCISION of OVARY, SKIN, PILONIDAL or other CYSTS?

Another example is the word MYCOSIS which means fungus disease, but in combination with FUNGOIDES means lymphoma of the skin. When a request for fungus disease was made, the search formulation excluded FUNGOIDES, that is, MYCOSIS not FUNGOIDES. In a search for lymphomas, however, the requester is asked whether he wants all lymphomas, and in one instance, the user wanted to exclude MYCOSIS FUNGOIDES and HODGKIN'S. This last request involved thought processes involving classification of diseases as well as just the meaning of the descriptor itself.

Combination of Descriptors (Not Multiple Word Descriptor)

The analyst views any combination of descriptors as representing a concept. For example, a request for all KIDNEY TRANSPLANT REJECTIONS will make the analyst think out loud that this request may need to include the descriptors INCOMPATIBILITY, GRAFT, DONOR, RECIPIENT, and can the requestor think of anything else? What about HOMOGRAFT? That descriptor is linked by the thesaurus to GRAFT. Then the relevant linkages in the thesaurus will be reviewed for verification by the requestor.

Multiple Searches By Creating Subsets

When a requestor submits several searches at the same time, the analyst sometimes can see a relationship between them, and when verified, analyzes the three searches as one concept. The retrieval is simplified by doing the most general part of the search first, creating subsets from the general matches, and performing separate retrievals from the subsets in one pass of the file. Printouts of data base reports can be produced after each step, or blanked out with only the total number of reports and patients appearing, according to his wishes.

Conceptual Differences Between Different Data Files

The same descriptors cannot be automatically used for each separate data base file. The procedures that are performed in each specialty and the way the findings are described vary and thus account for this difference. For example, a request for RHEUMATIC FEVER from the Surgical Pathology files would not be productive, while some cases may be retrieved from the Autopsy file. In one search, questioning revealed that the requestor was attempting to retrieve patients who had tissue removed at heart surgery. The request was modified to RHEUMATIC HEART and VALVE disease.

A request for thyroid malignancies from the several separate data bases cannot be satisfied by only searching for THYROID and MALIGNANCY. This search would be successful only for the pathology files. In addition, because we do not want to retrieve THYROID CARTILAGE from the pathology files, the request should be modified to THYROID not CARTILAGE. For searching the Nuclear Medicine file, the descriptors COLD or NONFUNCTIONING NODULE should be added to THYROID and MALIGNANCY in order to obtain all possible cases of thyroid malignancy in that file.

Current Terminology and Archaic Use of Terms

Medical science is dynamic, and the language used to describe disease conditions changes with time. Because the data base contains pathology reports accumulated since 1955, the analyst reflects upon how the data would be described in the old as well as the current data base. A search request for DOWN'S SYNDROME must include the descriptors MONGOLISM (old terminology) and TRISOMY-21 (recent terminology) as synonyms, and should be checked to make certain that these possible thesaurus linkages have been established in the thesaurus.

The People Concept (Human Factors)

Because the successful interactive session between requestor and analyst occurs only when human factors are taken into consideration, the analyst makes the system easy to use and accessible to the user. When a seemingly impossible request is made, instead of rejecting it, several alternatives are proposed to see if any of them would be acceptable. The system can furnish only information that is present in its data base, but with careful thought by the search analyst, it has been possible at times to produce acceptable results via an indirect mode when no other sources of data were available. The results may be a close estimate, and when it is, the requestor is asked to represent the findings that way rather than as a finite number.

If the physician has had success with past searches, he will have confidence in the system, and will participate with the analyst in obtaining the best results. Because it is thoroughly discouraging to be required to scan through unwanted material, the main purpose of the discussions is to remove as many irrelevant reports as possible without eliminating any of those that are relevant. The effective search analyst must recognize the limits of her knowledge and the need for dialogue with the requestor to clarify each search request before submitting it to the system. Experience has proved that when the requestor participates in the dialogue before complicated searches on submittal, he will be more satisfied with his retrieval than if he makes his request through the written form alone.

FORMULATING THE SEARCH

By the time the interactive session is completed, the analyst knows generally how the search will finally be formulated. Misspellings are corrected, the thesaurus is re-checked for linkages, the index of past search results is scanned for errors encountered in similar searches in the past, and reference books are checked to insure correct terminology for multiple word synonyms.

The requestor's intent, as determined by the interactive session, is then expressed as a search statement which often cannot be recognized as the original search request submitted by the user: one or more of the English terms may have been replaced by other descriptors or be in a different order, logical operators

may have been inserted between descriptors, search option symbols
may have been interposed, and in some instances, PL/1 coding may
have transformed the English search request into a statement that
looks like meaningless jargon to the requestor.

The conventional boolean algebraic operators of AND, OR, and
NOT are represented in the search statement with the symbols "&",
"|", and "⌐" respectively. The more terms that are ANDed together,
the more restrictive the search becomes. A search for POORLY &
DIFFERENTIATED & CARCINOMA will retrieve fewer cases than CARCINOMA.

The more logical alternatives that are expressed with OR
(|), the more documents will match the formulation. TUMOR &
(HEAD | NECK) will retrieve more documents than TUMOR & HEAD.

The use of negation or the logical NOT (⌐), can further
restrict a search to clarify any ambiguity of meaning where the
ambiguity is inherent in the word itself. WHIPPLE'S &⌐ DISEASE
will retrieve fewer cases than WHIPPLE'S alone. Because the
usage of the word WHIPPLE in surgical pathology refers more
frequently to WHIPPLE'S OPERATION, exclusion of WHIPPLE's DISEASE
which defines a different entity, will result in fewer false
positives when it is desired to retrieve data pertaining to this
surgical procedure. Cases containing both the word WHIPPLE'S and
WHIPPLE'S with the term OPERATION will be retrieved.

The NOT function is used to exclude a synonymous or subordinate term when it is not relevant for a particular search. The
logical NOT is also used to exclude specific descriptors which in
the context of a particular search may produce erroneous retrievals.

When negation of a whole synonym class or all the subordinate
classes contained in the thesaurus is needed, the search options
of NO SYNONYMS (#), NO SUBORDINATES ($), and WORD ONLY (# $) can
be used to suppress the usual complete structure search. Knowledge
of the thesaurus structure and word relationships assists the
analyst in making these decisions.

A few simple PL/1 programming codes allow age, sex, date, or
service restrictions to be added to the search when specified.
Such restrictions cause the testing of the appropriate fields on
the first identification and demographic record which heads each
of the reports in all the data files. Other fields that can be
tested are patient accession number, physician's name, bone
marrow, and financial information by departmental procedures in
the Surgical Pathology file; race, autopsy date, times of death
or autopsy, medical examiner status, and source of the request
for Autopsy in the Autopsy file.

Arithmetic operators used for testing these fields are:

=	Equal
⌐=	Not equal
>	Greater than
>=	Greater than or equal to
<	Less than
<=	Less than or equal to

ANALYSIS OF A SEARCH REQUEST

An illustration of the translation of the original written free
English request to the coded form follows:

SAMPLE SEARCH REQUEST: "Any tumor involving the orbit,
                           including the conjunctiva, eyelids,
                           and retro-orbital area classified
                           as lymphoma (Hodgkin's, non-Hodgkins's
                           lymphosarcoma, reticulum cell
                           sarcoma, or other) or abnormal
                           lymphocytic infiltration, diagnosed
                           in 1976." (Excluded mycosis fungoides
                           after questioning).

FORMULATED REQUEST: ((ORBIT ∣ EYE ⎸ EYELID) & ((LYMPHOMA
                           & ⌉ FUNGOIDES) ∣ (RETICULUM # $ &
                           SARCOMA $) ∣ (LYMPHOCYTIC & INFILTRA-
                           TION)))
                           % IF YR ⌉= '76" THEN RETURN (FALSE);

Analysis of this request reveals some of the modifications that
were made to perform this retrieval. Some linkages were already
present in the thesaurus: CONJUNCTIVA is subordinate to EYE,
RETRO-ORBITAL to ORBIT, and the different types of lymphomas
including MYCOSIS FUNGOIDES are subordinate to LYMPHOMAS. To
exclude MYCOSIS FUNGOIDES, only FUNGOIDES was excluded from the
subordinate classes below LYMPHOMA, because our experience with
past retrievals revealed FUNGOIDES always appeared with MYCOSIS.
RETICULUM has synonymous terms (RETICULAR, RETICULARIS) and a
subordinate class of terms (LYMPHORETICULAR); SARCOMA has subordinate classes of terms (OSTEOSARCOMA, ANGIOSARCOMA, CARCINOSARCOMA,
LIPOSARCOMA, etc.) that need not be represented in order to
obtain RETICULUM CELL SARCOMA. The word CELL was not included as
a search descriptor because our data base contains statements
that are worded RETICULUM SARCOMA (without CELL). Instead of
coding ABNORMAL with LYMPHOCYTIC INFILTRATION, all lymphocytic
infiltrations in the eye were retrieved for review, because
experience has shown that they are apt to be abnormal or at least
of interest to a requestor making this type of request.

THE SEARCH STRATEGY AND REPORT OPTIONS

The search programs locate all the documents in the data base
text files which have at least one representative descriptor
within a single diagnostic statement for each search descriptor.
A search through a report containing more than one diagnostic
statement continues through each segment of the diagnosis one at
a time until it finds a match or reaches the end of the report.
The patient identification number from a matching report is saved
in a HIT file which is then matched with the English text file
for printing of all of the patients' reports in chronological
order by date of procedure. As one of the report options, only
the reports that match the request can be printed, if this restriction is desired.

    Each list of retrieval documents routinely contains the
patient's identification number, last name and initials, age,
sex, accession number, date of procedure, and final diagnoses or
impressions.

Variety of Report Options

    The minimal information report option produces a single page
of the search printout with the total number of patients that
matched the search request, and total number of patients and
reports in file at time of the search. Retrievals of patient
medical record identification numbers only can also be obtained
by using the option for printing these numbers from the search's
HIT file. For demonstration purposes, the DEM option removes all
the patients' names from the printing to protect patient's right
of privacy. If a physician needs only a few cases, the MH (Maximum
Hits) option may be used to produce a specified number of cases.
"MH=25" will limit the search to a printing of twenty-five cases.

    Although most searches come under the category of routine
searches, a physician may want to search for the presence (or
absence) of an associated diagnosis (1) in another statement in
the same report, (2) in another report in the same data base, or
(3) in another report in a different Natural Language data base.

    In addition, the reports of the patient that meet the search
criteria from different data bases can be merged and printed in
chronological order. In some instances, the absence of a diagnosis
(or procedure) in the presence of another diagnosis (or procedure)
is of importance to a searcher. By using a NOHITS option, it is
possible to do a search for CERVICAL CONIZATIONS NOT FOLLOWED BY
HYSTERECTOMY, as well as CERVICAL CONIZATIONS FOLLOWED BY HYSTE-
RECTOMY. This option can be used in multiple data base searches
so that it is possible, for example to find patients with LIVER
SCANS HAVING NO LIVER BIOPSIES as well as LIVER SCANS HAVING
LIVER BIOPSIES.

Simple Multiple Data Base Match of Patients in Different Data Bases

    Since late 1975, every new group of completed surgical
pathology and autopsy reports has been matched with the other
Natural Language data bases of Nuclear Medicine and Neuroradiology
for the purpose of providing followup control on procedural and
reporting techniques for these departments. In 1977, bone marrow
reports were included in this routine matching with other data
bases. This match and merge function is only available in Natural
Language data bases.

Post-Retrieval

    Every search output is reviewed before delivery to the
requestor, so that false positives, if any, can be explained.
The physician may make suggestions which can be incorporated into
another search, if he wishes.

Data base errors detected by the search are noted and correction initiated. Those responsible for data entry and edit take note for future reference.

We have now reviewed the total concept of the system from data base to vocabulary to retrieval. All these elements of the system including the human factors are present in the thought processes of the search analyst during the discussions with the requestor. In a session that usually lasts less than fifteen minutes, the analyst can obtain enough information to produce a meaningful and accurate retrieval.

ON-LINE INTERACTION BEFORE RETRIEVAL

The question arises now as to how to facilitate the search process for the requester with a preplanned device or mechanism that is able to mimic the behavior or performance of the human interface, that is, in principle, fully predictable. An important class of artificial intelligence devices is the kind that is the adaptive or the learning type, which modifies its behavior with acquired experience through trial and error. These devices sometimes surpass the performance of their designers, but can only learn and adapt in the manner or degree set forth by the designers. Admittedly, many cognitive processes cannot now be imitated by the computer, such as perception and creative insight which involve extremely complicated interplay of the mind and the senses in producing subjective images of complex phenomena.

It should be possible in the on-line use of our natural language system to program straightforward search logic during a portion of the interactive session. The interrogation process should be simple with a reasonable amount of steps and enough on-line prompting and choices so that steps can be skipped if the searcher desires. Errors in spelling should be quickly identified and easy to correct. Response time should not be too long or the search formulation too complex for the requester's tolerance and span of attention.

Some sequential decision-making may be accomplished by routine questions presently requested on the request form such as: searcher's name, department, and phone number; data bases to be searched; kind of search; maximum number of documents requested; and the reason for the search; however, the nuances of some of the answers to these questions may be lost.

The problems become obviously more difficult when analyzing how the computer will help express the request in coded form from an initial free form search request.

Medical researchers would probably prefer the heuristic process of the interactive on-line search. The searcher can try various term combinations, review records that match these strategies, examine the terms, and revise his strategy based on a selection of pertinent terms using vocabulary displays.

Some aids that would be advantageous to the searcher would be the ability to browse through selected parts of the thesaurus with updated frequency counts for terms and an easy way of referencing synonymous multiple word descriptors and logical relations, which are complex network structures of cross linkages combining two or more synonym classes to represent another search entity. This browsing would assist him in obtaining the desired level of specificity for each search descriptor. The searcher's attention can then be directed to prefixes (EXTRA-, PARA-, besides the others previously mentioned) and parts of speech (adjective form of the word root; adverbs, and prepositions) that transform the site to an adjacent structure or geographic area so that he can indicate the inclusion or exclusion of these terms in his request.

The most difficult part would be to recall all the characteristics of the data base file content, the differences as well as the similarities, and to provide the imagination necessary for developing acceptable alternative suggestions for something not directly obtainable. The decisions on how to combine all the knowledge and experience with the system of the system designers and defining the interaction with different searchers while evaluating their answers in a conversational mode present a further challenge to the designer of an on-line interface to the present natural language system.

New design concepts must be employed and the tendency to take an existing batch-processing system and merely make the data base available on-line is not the best approach. In addition to being highly desirable, natural language systems are becoming increasingly feasible because digital storage costs are decreasing with the development of mass storage devices of various types, and machine-readable data bases will be available as by-products of other operations. In conclusion, the on-line interactive mode of operation must be designed with the needs of the searcher and department users, not the information analyst, primarily in mind. We contemplate proceeding along these lines in the near future.

REFERENCE

R.S. Okubo, W.S. Russel, B. Dimsdale and B.G. Lamson, Natural Language Storage and Retrieval of Medical Diagnostic Information, Computer Programs in Biomedicine, 5 (1975), 105-130.

Computational Linguistics in Medicine, Schneider/Sagvall Hein, eds.
North-Holland Publishing Company, (1977)

MORPHOSYNTACTICAL ANALYSIS OF MEDICAL COMPOUND WORD FORMS

F. WINGERT

Institut für Medizinische Informatik und Biomathematik,
Universität Münster, Westdeutschland

A model for segmentation of German or English compound word forms and its implementation is described. Components of the model are (1) segment dictionary, with 10.415 English and German segments, (2) a rule system with 256 rules in a hierarchical graph notation and (3) an algorithm for segmentation.

1 INTRODUCTION

The model has emerged from former research. Results have been published |3| and will only be mentioned if they are necessary for understanding.

Morphological analysis of compound word forms is done here to facilitate semantical analysis of a medical utterance formulated in medical language |4|. So far, it is a technical tool which serves for reduction of size and update frequency of the dictionary. The possibility for logical deduction and the independence of the special "mother language" make it a powerful tool.

Compound word forms are constructed in a fairly regular way by concatenation of "segments". The set of all segments can be broken down into disjoint subsets, each subset playing a different role with respect to semantics, syntactics and translation from one mother language to another. One first version of the model |3| has been extended to the segmentation of the suffixes. The results are a slight increase in ambiguity and complexity and a significant decrease in the number of segments and update frequency.

The system has been developed as a subsystem for automatic indexing of medical diagnoses. It has been devised with regard to independence from the special "mother language" English or German |4| . For indexing purposes the Systematized Nomenclature of Pathology (SNOP |1|,|2|) has been chosen but the algorithms are independent of the special thesaurus.

2 SEGMENTATION

Systems for analysis of language data are faced with several problems:

- The dictionary sizes create problems in storage and retrieval. Therefore, methods for reduction of dictionary size have to be looked for to avoid as far as possible the necessity of formulating the utterance in artificial languages using a reduced vocabulary.

- Missing algorithms for semantical analysis of utterances in (nearly) natural language have to be compensated by dictionaries listing semantically ordered data atoms. These data atoms should be defined semantically and should be based on segments. If they are based on words, then a high degree of redundancy is created by the significant number of compound words. Rules have to be developed for the decomposition of the utterances into data atoms.

The advantages of a sophisticated segmentation procedure are:

- The size of the segment dictionary is given by the sum of the numbers of different segment types, whereas the size of a full word dictionary is in the magnitude of the product of the numbers of the different components.

- Medical language is a living language and new words are generated mostly by construction of new compound words using well-known segments.

- About 2/3 of medical segments are language independent, i.e., they are of either Latin or Greek origin (see table 3). In full words they are often inflected in a language dependent manner.

The term "segment" corresponds to the linguistic entity "morpheme". Differences are based on the fact, that not only linguistics but also efficiency of the algorithm has been considered. Moreover, segmentation which goes too far-due to semantic criteria - (e.g. EPI|PHYSIS) is compromised by the thesaurus used for indexing.

2.1 Word model

Segmentation presupposes a word model. The model determines dictionary size to such a degree that as far as possible it should reflect the linguistic principles of construction of a word. For instance, if words can be defined as productions of different types of components, then dictionary size is reduced most when all the components are broken down into disjoint sets and when the number of sets is a maximum.

A word w is a sequence of word parts v_i:

$$w = v_1 v_2 \ldots v_k, \tag{1}$$

and each word part is a sequence of a root (r) and a suffix. The empty string is a suffix. A suffix consists of a derivational suffix (s) and a terminal suffix (t). Therefore, the word model is:

$$w = \underbrace{r_1 s_1 t_1}_{v_1} \underbrace{r_2 s_2 t_2}_{v_2} \ldots \underbrace{r_k s_k t_k}_{v_k} \quad (k \geq 1). \tag{2}$$

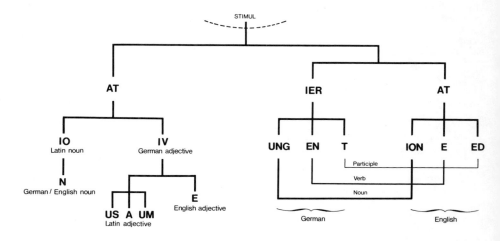

Fig. 1: Corresponding families of suffixes for a class of roots (e.g., STIMUL)

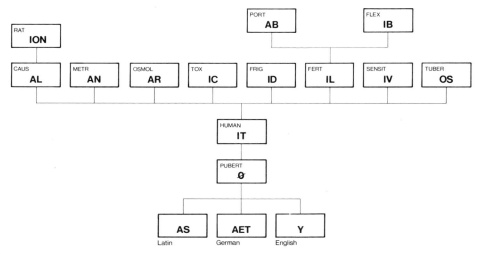

Fig. 2: Hierarchical relations between suffix families (read top down). Each node
corresponds to a family which can be concatenated to a class of roots.
Each set is represented by one element. The "leaves" represent a set of
inflectional suffixes

Terminal suffixes $t_1, t_2, \ldots, t_{k-1}$ are connectors, terminal suffix t_k is an inflectional suffix. Each s_i and/or t_i may be the empty string, no r_i can be
the empty string (i=1,2,...,k).

Suffixes can be looked at as families (see fig. 1) which are connected to each
other (see fig. 2). The composition of families has several advantages, because
many noun/adjectival transformations and translations (e.g., between English,
German and Latin) are done by exchange of suffixes or just exchange of terminal
suffix.

The basic idea of word segmentation is to determine the sets of derivational suffixes succeeding to a special root, the sets of terminal suffixes succeeding to a
special derivational suffix, and which word parts can be at the beginning, within
or at the end of a word. Additionally, there has to be an algorithm for the determination of the best choice, if for a given word w and for a given segment μ more
than one successor is possible. These determinations are done by a set of <u>rules</u>,
and the <u>principle   of longest match</u>.

2.2   Definitions

2.2.1 Lists

A string consists of a finite number of alphabetic and/or numeric characters. The
empty string is denoted by $\emptyset$. Two strings μ_1 and μ_2 may be concatenated to string
$\mu = \mu_1 \, \mu_2$. Two strings μ_1 and μ_2 hold the relation $\mu_1 < \mu_2$, if μ_2 succeeds to μ_1 in
alphabetic order.

A <u>simple list</u> is a set of strings:

$$\ell = \mu_1, \, \mu_2, \ldots, \mu_k. \tag{3}$$

If ℓ is a simple list (see eq. (3)) and μ is a string, then the product $\mu(\ell)$ is defined as the set:

$$\mu(\ell) = \mu(\mu_1, \mu_2, \ldots, \mu_k) = \mu\mu_1, \mu\mu_2, \ldots, \mu\mu_k. \qquad (4)$$

A <u>list</u> is a set of products between strings μ_i and lists ℓ_i

$$\ell = \mu_1(\ell_1), \mu_2(\ell_2), \ldots, \mu_k(\ell_k). \qquad (5)$$

2.2.2 Rules

A rule

$$n\, L_n = x_n; y_n \qquad (6)$$

consists of the identifying number n, the language marker L_n, the morphological expression x_n and the syntactical/semantical information y_n (see table 1). The <u>identifying number</u> n ($0 \leq n \leq 255$) is used for reference. The <u>language marker</u> L_n denotes the language the rule belongs to (/ for German, $\emptyset$ for English and & for German and English). If the position of the language marker is empty, then it has to be derived from the morphological expression x_n (see below).

A <u>morphological expression</u> x_n is a list connected to syntactical/semantical information y_n ("connected to y_n"). A morphological expression defines a set of suffixes, e.g., inflectional suffixes of German adjectives: $x_n = ,E(,M,N,R,S)$.

<u>Syntactical informations</u> refer to language, part of speech, word part and gender (see table 2). They can be used later for syntactical analysis of utterances.

The most important <u>semantical informations</u> are the positions with respect to the thesaurus used (SNOP-codes $\boxed{1}$, $\boxed{2}$). If there is an equivalence between a morphological expression x_n and SNOP-codes, then these SNOP-codes are listed following the character '$*$' (e.g., rule 183 for inflammations, see table 1). Additional syntactical/semantical informations are in table 2.

The use of <u>hierarchical ordered graphs</u> is made possible by the definitions given in section 2.2.1: If the morphological expression x_n of a rule n corresponding to z_n contains the morphological expression x_m of a rule m corresponding to y_m, and if x_m implies the subset $y_m \subset z_n$,

$$m\, L_m = x_m; y_m$$
$$n\, L_n = x_n^{(o)}, \mu(x_m), x_n^{(1)}; z_n, \; z_n = y_n \cup y_m,$$

then rule n can be written as

$$n\, L_n = x_n^{(o)}, \mu(m), x_n^{(1)}; y_n.$$

In this formula, the explicitly listed syntactical/semantical information can be reduced. From now, the complete syntactical/semantical information (no implicit informations) of a rule n will be denoted as y_n^*. In analogy, the language marker is derived, if it is not given explicitly: If there is at least one reference and if all references have the same language marker, then this language marker is attached to the rule, else the language marker & is attached to the rule.

Example (see table 1): If rule 219 and 89 respectively had come to be

219/ = ,E(,M,N,R,S); D ADJ   89/ = AER (,E(,M,N,R,S)); D ADJ

then finally rule 89 is written as: 89 = AER(219);

Corresponding to the relation between x_n and y_n, a morphological expression has to be <u>resolved</u>. If a reference j in a rule i is substituted by x_j, then the syntactical/semantical information y_i has to be replaced by the union $y_i \cup y_j$. Therefore two morphological expressions x_i and x_j are equivalent, when and only when there is a sequence of substitutions which transform x_i into x_j or vice versa and when $y_i^* = y_j^*$.

Table 1: Rules (Notation see section 2.2.2)

```
 1/=L(19);
 2 =-;                              ABK
 3 =A(,238,255,T(253));             G L D N
 4 =I( 54);
 5 =AUE(242,255);
 6 =AT(20V,241),A( 55),203;         L D E F
 7 =AGE(242,255);
 8 =AI(I 39),KI 39));
 9 =ASM( 3,255);
10 =AT( 14,234,237);                N M
11 =AT( 46);
12 =AT( 61);
13 =CHEN(238),LET(255);             N
14 =E(223,235,238,242,255);
15 =E(249);
16 =EL(235,242,255),L( 14);
17 =ELL( 14, 48, 52,226,248);       F M
18 =EN,IN(253);                     N M
19 =EK(235,255);
20 =EK(252,253),R(252);
21 =HEIT(20V,241),NESS(254);        F
22 =I( 14,226,248,A(,255)),203;     ALLG F
23 =I( 14,226,248,A(,255)),203;     KRANKH GATTG F
24 =I( 54);
25 =I(232,249);
26 =I(231);                         N
27 =IAS( 14,22V);                   F
28 =IC(232,241,249,255);
29 =ICI 39);
30 =I( 25,214,225,226,234,248,249,E(242));  GATTG ALLG
31 =IDI 39);
32 =ILI 14, 25,225,234);            CHEM ALLG N
33 =IL( 39);
34/=IN(,N(241));
35 =IN( 39);
36 =I0(,N(20V,241,252,255));        F
37 =IONAL( 39);
38 =IT( 14,237);                    ALLG M N
39 =IT( 6);
40 =IV( 39);
41 =I(X,C(252));
42 =KE,I(20V,241);
43/=LING(20V,234);                  M
44/=NIS(,SE(,S,N));                 N F
45 =0(241),IN(252),UN(252);
46 =0U(228,248,E(242));             GATTG G D M
47 =0ID(234,255);                   M
48 =0ID(228,248);
49 =OL( 14,214,226,233,247,248,249);  ALLG
50 =OM( 3,234);                     N ALLG
51 =OK(236,252,255);
52 =OS( 14,22V);                    KRANKH ALLG F
53 =US( 39);
54 =S,O(206,214,230,252);
55 =S,T(221,252);
56 =SCHAFT(20V,241);
57 =UL( 14,247);                    M
58 =ULI 14,248);                    F
59 =UL( 14,24V);                    N
60 =UNG(20V,241);
61 =UK( 14,241,248);                F
62 =UR(253),OK(253);
63 =US,EK(253),OK(253);             N F
64 =U(X,C(252));
65 =X,G(252);
663=EU( 21);
673=M0U0;
683=IVE( 21);
69 =AL(225,234,249,255);            CHEM ALLG N
70 =AN( 14,234,249);                CHEM N
71 =AS( 14);                        ENZ F
72 =AT( 14,234);                    SALZ N
73 =EN( 14, 25,234);                CHEM N
74 =ID( 14, 25,214,234);            SALZ N
75 =IO( 71);
76 =IN( 14, 25,214,234,249,255);    CHEM N
77 =IN( 71);
78 =IT( 14,214,234);                SALZ N
79 =OL( 14, 25,234,249);            ALKOHOL N
80 =OL( 71);
81 =ON( 14, 25,214,234);            KETON ALLG N
82 =OS( 14,22V);                    ZUCKEK F
83 =YL( 25,234,249);                CHEM N
84 =YL( 71);
85 =+,S,I(,I);                      NAME ALLG
86 =AC( 96);
87 =AL(145,219,221);
88 =AL(108);
89 =AK(103,130,219,221),8K(219);
90 =AK(103,130,219),8K(219);
91 =AT(129,214,219,220);            PP ADJ L D
92 =AT(108);
93 =AT(115);
94 =AT(116);
95 =AT(121);
96 =E( 14,201,220,247,248);
97 =E( 67);
983=I(129);
99/=E,L(219);
100 =EN,S(,221);
101 =EK(,220),R(221,220);
102/=PACH(,219);
103 =I(220,233,247);
104 =I( 87);
105 =I( 87, 90);
106 =I( 91);
107 =I( 97);
108 =I(C(, 87,214,220),SCH(219),QUE);
109 =U(214,219,220);
110 =I(214,219,221);
111 =IN(129,214,219,221);
112 =ION( 87);
113 =ION( 89);
114 =ION( 99);
115 =IV(129,219,220,226,234,248,249);
116 =OU(214,219);
117 =OIU( 46);
118 =OID( 87);
11V =U( 92);
120 =U(103,130,203,I(232,249));
121 =U(108);
122a=OUS;
122a=OU(214,220),+S(219);
123 =UT(108);
124a=TH;                            I/A0
124=T(219);                         URU
125 =U(214,220);
126 =UL( 89, 90);
127 =UL( 91);
128 =UL( 122);
129$=E;
130a=Y;
131a=EU(X,SE);
```

```
132$=EK;                            KOM
132 =EK(219);                       KOM
133 =I(134);
134 =UK(219,252),US;                KOM
135a=EST;                           SUP
135/=EST(219),ST(219);              SUP
136 =I,SI(M(220);                   SUP
137/=-;                             KJG U
138&=,E(,S);                        VR8
139&=,S;                            VR8
140&=,EU;                           PP
140/=ET(219);                       PP
141&=ING;                           PPK
142&=N;                             PP
143 =,E;                            ADV
144/=S;                             ADV
145 =L(130);                        ADV
146 =-;                             CAR
147 =-;                             KJK
148 =-;                             NEG
149 =-;                             PRÄF
150 =-;                             ASS
151 =-;                             PRN
152 =-;                             PRP
153 =-;                             ZIF
154 =,SCH(219),S,I(,I),201,202;     EPO
155 =AL( 96,IL( 39,221));
156 =AL(I(B));
157 =AN( 39, 96,108,219,220);
158 =AN(S,T( 22, 25,104,107,145,219,221,237,255),Z(175,241),C( 14,203));
159 =AT( 36,138,140,141),175;
160 =AT( 51,120,121);
161 =AT( 52,122,123);
162 =AIX,C(221,252));
163 =BAK( 42,219);
164 =EN( 3, 92, 94,108,161,234,255,ATIS(175));
165/=,EN(,U(21V)),T( 21,219);       INF PTZ
166 =EN( 21,21V);                   PP
167 =EN(S,T( 22, 25,104,107,145,219,221,237,255),Z(175,241),C( 14,203));
168/=EK( 60,188,206);
169 =EI(S( 14,22V),T(108));
170$=ESC(138,140,141,ENC( 14));
170&=ES(CENIS,T(221)),CIEKE(188),ZENZ(241));
171 =EX,C(221,252);
172 =I( 52,123);
173 =IAI( 96,IL( 39,221));
174 =ICAN(S,T(219,221),Z(241),C( 14));
175&=AT(ION(255),138,140,141));
175/=EN( 60,163,165);
176 =IG( 60,165);
177/=IG( 42,219);
178 =IL(18(21);
179 =IL(182);
180 =IUN(140,141,175);
181&=IZ(AT(ION(255),138,140,141);
181&=IS(138,140,141,159,AT(220));
182 =IS(M(233,247,255),T(108));
183 =IT( 24,108),M4000
184/=IL( 60),EL( 60,188,206);
185 =LICH( 42, 60,219);
186&=LESS( 21,219);
186/=LOS(219,IG( 42));
187 =MENT( 87, 89,234,249,255);
188 =N(238,0(219)),T(219);          INF PTZ
189 =OID(182);
190 =OID(183);
191 =OID(183);
192 =OM( 3, 94,161,234);            MED ALLG
193 =OS(175);
194 =OS(183);
195/=SAM( 42,219);
196 =ULAN(S,T(219,221,237),Z(241),C( 14));
197 =UL(159);
198 =UL(183);
19V =UL( 52,116,122,123);
200/=KTISCH(219);
200&=XI( 22),CT(108);
201&=AN;                            ADJ
202&=I(201);
203&=Y,I,IES;                       SUB
204 =-;                             FIN
205 =-;                             ART
206 =-;                             FUG
207 =-;                             FUG
208/=EN;                            FUG
209/=S;                             FUG
210 =-;                             FUG
211 =E(214);
212 =I;                             FUG
213 =I(214);
214 =0(216);                        FUG
215 =0(216);                        FUG
216 =R;                             FUG
217 =Y;                             FUG
218 =-;                             INT
219&=;                              E ADJ AOV
219/=,E(,M,N,S,R);                  D ADJ
220$=0US;                           ADJ
220&=U(S,M),I(,S),0(,RUM),A(,E,M,S,KUM);  ADJ L
221 =,E(,M,S),I(,I,A,S,UM,BUS),UM;  ADJ L
222 =,E(,S),S;                      SIT
223 =,N;                            PLT
224/=EN;                            PLT
225&=,S,I(224);                     SUB GRM N
226&=A,224;                         SUB GRM N
227&=A(,S),224;                     SUB GRM N
228 =E(,IS;                         SUB GATTG G M KRANKH L F
229 =I(S,N);                        SUB G F
230 =I(S,N);                        SUB G N
231&=ON(,S),I,A,224;                SUB G D GRM N M
232&=UM(,S),224;                    SUB GRM N
233&=U(S,224);                      SUB GRM M N
234/=,S,E(,S,N);                    SUB M N
235/=,S,N;                          SUB M N
236/=,S,E(,S,N);                    SUB M N
237/=,EN;                           SUB M
238/=,S,E(,S);                      SUB M N
239/=,E(,N(,S));                    SUB N N
240/=,E(,N);                        SUB F
241/=,EN,NEN;                       SUB F
242/=,N;                            SUB N
243/=,S,E(,S,R(,N));                SUB GRM M F N
244 =,S;                            SUB F
245 =E(S,I);                        SUB L E
246 =U(,S,M,UM);                    SUB L K N F
247 =U(S,M),I(,S),O(,RUM);          SUB M L
248 =A(,E,M,RUM,S),IS;              SUB L F GATTG
249 =UM,I(,S),O(,RUM),A;            SUB L N F
250 =I(,S,UM,BUS),E(,M,S);          SUB L M F
251 =E,I(,A,BUS,S,UM);              SUB L N
252 =,I(,S,BUS,UM),E(M,S,UM);       SUB L M F
253 =I(,A,S,UM),A,UM;               SUB L N
254&=,ES;                           SUB
255&=,S;                            SUB
```

Table 2: Syntactical/semantical informations

Syntactical informations:

Language		word part	
L	Latin	PRF	Prefix
G	Greek	ASS	Prefix, assimilated
D	German	FUG	Connector
GRM	Germanized	FIN	Segment, not last in a word
E	English		

Parts of speech

VRB	Verb	ADJ	Adjective
PTZ	Participle	KOM	Comparative
PPR	Present participle	SUP	Superlative
PP	Past participle	CAR	Cardinalium
INF	Infinitive	ORD	Ordinalium
KJG	Conjuncted form	PRN	Pronoun
SUB	Noun	PAR	Particle
EPO	Eponym	ADV	Adverb
INT	Interimistic form	KJK	Conjunction
SIT	Singularetantum	PRP	Preposition
PLT	Pluraletantum	ABK	Abbreviation
ART	Article	ZIF	Numeral
DET	Definite article		
IDT	Indefinite article		

Semantical informations:

ALLG	General segment	SALZ	Salt
GATTG	Generic name	ALKOHOL	Alcohol
CHEM	Chemical	KETON	Ketone
KRANKH	Disease	ZUCKER	Sugar
MED	Medical term	NAME	Name
ENZ	Encyme	NEG	Negation

If, for instance, rule j is

$$j \ L_j = x_j; y_j,$$

then the following notations for rule i are equivalent:

$$i \ L_i = \mu_i(j); y_i$$
$$i \ L_i = \mu_i(x_j); y_i \cup y_j.$$

This notation has the advantages of a formal language, e.g.,

- Low redundancy.

- Language marker, list and syntactical/semantical information have to be listed
  explicitly only in case they cannot be derived from the morphological expression. Therefore, alterations in the system of rules can be done with minimal
  changes which is of high value during development.

- The dictionaries of suffixes can be generated automatically (see section 2.3.3).

2.3   Word segmentation

2.3.1 Usage of rules

After resolution of all references in x_n, x_n is a set of strings (suffixes),
$x_n = \mu_1, \mu_2, \ldots, \mu_k$. For instance (see table 1):

x_{94} = AT(116) = AT(OID(214,219)) = AT(OID(O,,E(,M,N,R,S))) =
= ATOIDO, ATOID, ATOIDE, ATOIDEM, ATOIDEN, ATOIDER, ATOIDES.

If a root r may have all these suffixes, i.e., if all the products (see eq. (4)):

$$r\ (x_n) = r\ \mu_1,\ r\ \mu_2,\dots,r\ \mu_k$$

are word parts with a syntactical/semantical information which is a superset to y_n, then "rule n applies to root r". If suffix μ belongs to x_n, then "rule n applies to suffix μ". For instance, rule 94 may apply to root RHEÚM. Then the strings RHEU-MATOIDO, RHEUMATOID,... are word parts.

To break suffixes down into derivational suffixes and terminal suffixes, two disjoint sets of identifying numbers are defined: Numbers between 0 and 204 define rs-products, numbers between 205 and 255 define rɸt- and st-products.

(1) For n< 205, x_n may be resolved such, that x_n contains those and only those references≥205. Then x_n may be written as

$$x_n = \mu_1,\dots,\ \mu_i,\ \mu_{i+1}(n_{i+1}),\dots,\ \mu_k(n_k),\ n_j \geq 205;\ j = i+k,\dots,k.$$

If rule n applies to root r and s = μ_j, then each pair <rs> is a valid pair, if rule n applies to segment s, i.e., j≤k.

Furthermore, every product <rsɸ> is a word part, if j≤i.

For a derivational suffix μ_j not only rule n, but also rule n_j (j = i+1,...,k) applies. This is the way to connect both types of suffixes (see below).

For instance (see table 1):

$$x_{133}= I(134) = I(OR(219,252),US) = IOR(219,252),IUS.$$
$$\mu_1 = IUS,\ \mu_2 = \mu_3 = IOR,\ n_2 = 219,\ n_3 = 252.$$

Rule 133 may apply to root INFER. Then the string INFERIOR is a valid pair <rs> and the string INFERIUS is a word part <rsɸ> .

(2) For n≥205, all references in x_n may be resolved. Then x_n may be written as a simple list (see eq. (3)).

If rule n applies to root r resp. derivational suffix s, then each product <rɸt> is a word part resp. <st> is a valid pair, if rule n applies to segment t, i.e., t∈ x_n. If rule n applies to terminal suffix t, then t∈ x_n.

For instance, rule 231 (see table 1) may apply to root PARADOX. Then the string PARADOXON is a word part <rɸt> .

In addition to the special cases s = ∅ or t = ∅ there is: A string <rst> is a word part, if there applies at least one rule n< 205 to r and s and at least one rule m≥205 to s and t. For instance (for the identifying numbers see table 1):

<rst> = ACANTH   OS   IS ,   <rɸt>= HEPAT   O...(GASTRICUM),
              ⌣   ⌣   ⌣
              52   229   214

<rsɸ> = REN   AL... ,   <rɸɸ> = NEPHR ...   (ECTOMY).
            ⌣   ⌣   ⌣
            87   221   206

2.3.2 Word parts

There are 5 additional prescriptions concerning concatenation of word parts (see eq. (1)) which can be partly derived from the rules:

(1) $v_1,v_2,\dots,v_{k-1}$ may not be the terminal word part.

(2) v_k may be the terminal word part (e.g.,last segment not a connector, rule 204 does not apply).

(3) For k >1, for no word part v_i a rule applies which indicates that v_i can never be connected with another segment (e.g.,rules 2 and 205).

(4) At most 3 prefixes (rule 149 or 150 applies to a root) can be connected with each other.

(5) If a prefix has length 1, then the succeeding character must be a consonant.

Following this the definition of a valid sequence of segments can be derived, which is needed for the segmentation algorithm (see section 2.3.3.2):

$\mu_1\mu_2...\mu_i$ is a <u>valid sequence of segments</u>, if the string μ_j μ_{j+1} is a valid pair or if μ_j is the last segment of a word part and μ_{j+1} is a root ($j=1,2,...,i-1$) and rules (1) to (5) hold.

2.3.3 Implementation

2.3.3.1 Dictionaries

3 dictionaries are necessary for segmentation, i.e., dictionary of roots, derivational suffixes and terminal suffixes (see table 3). The structure of an element of one of these dictionaries is

$$\text{<type> <}\mu\text{> L } i_1 i_2 ... i_k \left[\text{<SNOP-codes>} \right] .$$

<type> indicates the segment type (R for roots, S for derivational suffixes and T for terminal suffixes). L is the language marker and i_j are the identifying numbers of those rules which apply to the segment ($j = 1,2,...,k$). If there is an equivalent for a segment μ in SNOP, then the respective SNOP-codes are listed.

Examples: (T1131 △ CLAVICULA)

<type>	<μ>	L	i_1	i_2	...	i_k	
R	CLAVIC	&	16	58		126	T1131
S	UL	&	57	58...248		249	
S	ULAR	&	126	219		221	
T	A	&	210	220	...	248	
T	IS	&	220	221	...	253	

Following section 2.3.1 there is:

(1) <type> = R

  <rs> = $\mu\mu_1$ is a valid pair resp. <røt> = $\mu\mu_1$ is a word part, if at least one rule i_j applies for μ_1, $i_j <$ 205 for <rs> resp. $i_j \geq$ 205 for <røt> . For instance: μ = CLAVIC, μ_1 = UL, <rs> = CLAVICUL (i_j = 58).

(2) <type> = S

  (2.1) <rs> = $\mu_1\mu$ is a valid pair (see (1)).

  (2.2) <st> = $\mu\mu_1$ is a valid pair if at least one rule i_j applies for μ_1, $i_j \geq$ 205.

  For instance: μ = UL, μ_1 = A, <st> = ULA (i_j = 248).

(3) <type> = T

  (3.1) <st> = $\mu_1\mu$ is a valid pair (see (2.2)).

  (3.2) <røt> = $\mu\mu_1$ is a word part (see (1)).

For instance: <rst> = CLAVICULA and <rst> = CLAVICULARIS are word parts.

The dictionaries of suffixes can be generated automatically by resolution of the rule system (see table 1).For a better overwiew the graph corresponding to rule families can be plotted (see fig. 3,4).

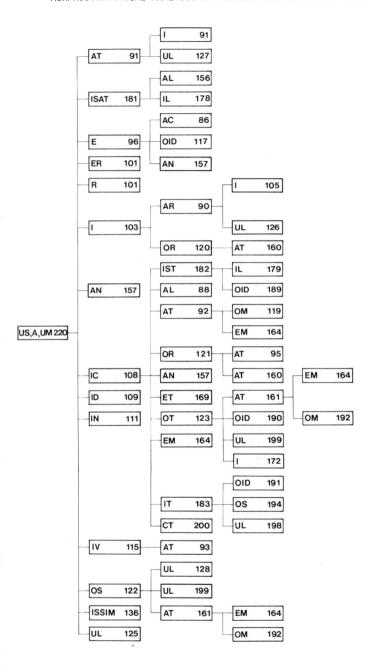

Fig. 3: Hierarchical graph of all families of suffixes referencing rule 220

Segments and rules cover more than 100.000 word parts (German language). The number of medical words which can be analyzed is by far greater than this figure. A summary of the contents of the dictionaries is given in Table 3.

If there are graphemic variants due to C-K-Z-exchange then only the C-variant is taken into the dictionary. The variants are also handled by the algorithm.

2.3.3.2 Segmentation Algorithm

The segmentation algorithm emerges from the definitions given above. If there is a sequence

$$w = \mu_1 \mu_2 \cdots \mu_{i-1} \mu_i X$$

consisting of a valid sequence of segments and remainder X, then the longest segment μ_{i+1} is looked up, such that there is a valid sequence of segments and remainder Y:

$$w = \mu_1 \mu_2 \cdots \mu_{i-1} \mu_i \mu_{i+1} Y.$$

If such a segment is found and Y is not the empty string, the algorithm proceeds. If such a segment is not found, then it is proved, whether there is a segment σ_i, resulting in a valid sequence of segments with remainder Z:

$$w = \mu_1 \mu_2 \cdots \mu_{i-1} \sigma_i Z, \ \sigma_i < \mu_i.$$

If such a segment σ_i is found, the algorithm proceeds. If such a segment σ_i is not found, μ_{i-1} is replaced. The algorithm stops, when the word is either completely segmentated; i.e.,

$$w = \mu_1 \mu_2 \cdots \mu_k$$

is a valid sequence of segments or there is no μ_1 found. In the latter case, all letters K and Z in the word are replaced permutatively by letter C and after each replacement segmentation is tried again.

The 3 dictionaries are loaded as compressed binary trees. Total space needed is 97 KBytes. Time tests for the 12.000 different words of German SNOP |2| resulted in an average of 2.5 msec/word on an IBM/370-168.

The rate of semantically incorrect segmentations is about 1 % related to 12.000 (different) words of German SNOP |2| (e.g., MY   O   P   I   A   instead of

$\qquad\qquad\qquad\qquad\qquad\qquad\quad r_1 \quad t_1 \quad r_2 \quad s_2 \quad t_2$

MY   OP   I   A).

$r_1 \quad r_2 \quad s_2 \quad t_2$

In most cases the more efficient way of correction is the use of some longer segment which avoids wrong segmentation based on principle of longest match (e.g.,MYOP) instead of changes to the algorithm or to the rules.

Table 3: Contents of the Dictionaries

The dictionaries of suffixes are generated automatically from the rules (see table 1)

Segment type	German	English	German/English	Total
Root	1844	961	6794	9599
Derivational suffix	209	316	241	766
Terminal suffix	23	1	26*	50
Total	2076	1278	7061	10415

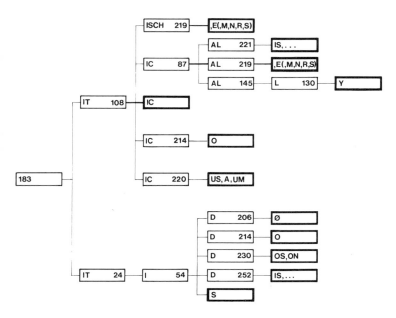

Fig. 4: Hierarchical graph of all references of rule 183

ACKNOWLEDGEMENT:

Several colleagues helped me in doing the technical work. Special thanks has to be given to Henning Siebel for his valuable help in updating the rule system.

REFERENCES:

1   College of American Pathologists: Systematized Nomenclature of Pathology
     Chicago: 1969

2   Wingert, F. and P. Graepel: Systematized Nomenclature of Pathology
     Deutsche Übersetzung
     Schriftenreihe des Instituts für Medizinische Informatik und Biomathematik,
     Nr. 1, Münster, 1975

3   Wingert, F.: Word Segmentation and Morpheme Dictionary for Pathology Data
     Processing
     In: Anderson, J. and J. Forsythe: MEDINFO 74, North-Holland Publ. Comp.: 1975

4   Wingert, F.: Medical Language Data Processing
     In: Reichertz, P.L., Goos, G.: Informatics and Medicine
     Berlin, Heidelberg, New York: Springer 1977

Computational Linguistics in Medicine, Schneider/Sågvall Hein, eds.
North-Holland Publishing Company, (1977)

AN APPROACH TO
THE CONSTRUCTION OF A TEXT COMPREHENSION SYSTEM
FOR X-RAY REPORTS

Anna-Lena Sågvall Hein
Uppsala University Data Center
Uppsala, Sweden

An attempt to design and build a teachable text comprehension
system for a given subdomain is described. The sample texts are
authentic x-ray examination reports on medial collum fractures
in the hip. Analyzing a set of reports the system is supposed
to build up a knowledge base about the subject matter being
described. At the beginning of the learning process, i e when
the analysis of the first sentence of the first report is started,
the system has a dictionary, a grammar and a few assumptions
about the text linguistic structure at its disposal. Semantic
relations between conceptual words are substituted for syntactic
constituents, recognized during the parsing process. The parser
works within the chart-analysis framework suggested by Kay (see ref).

INTRODUCTION

When a person reads and understands a text he makes use not only of his knowledge
about the language in which the text is written but also of his knowledge about
the subject matter. A major problem in modelling the process of text comprehension
in the computer is to decide on what knowledge is required and how it should be
represented and referenced. The aim of this work is to gain some insight into
these problems, and, mainly, to see how far we could get in building up the necessary knowledge base automatically. I work with a set of authentic x-ray examination reports on medial collum fractures in the hip, where, basically, the
same reality is described in many different ways.

GENERAL STRATEGY

Basically, I work with the idea that the syntactic relations between the linguistic units - the words within the sentence and the sentences within the report -
reflect conceptual relations which can be used in building a semantic representation. Semantic relations between conceptual words are substituted for syntactic
constituents recognized during the parsing procedure. This substitution is succes-
sively carried out as the constituents are found, i e as the result of the parsing
we don't get a syntactic but a semantic tree. For an illustration, let us look at
fig 1.

The string 'Medial collumfraktur, som är inkilad.' is recognized by the parser as
a sentence, consisting of a nominal phrase with 'fraktur' as its head. 'fraktur'
is specified in two ways, by the first component 'collum' in the compound 'collumfraktur' and by the relative clause. 'collum' is specified by the attribute 'medial'. The syntactic relation (ATTR NOUN) and (NOUN REL_CLAUSE) and the lexical
relation between the two components in the compound correspond in this system to
a subordination relation. I distinguish between different types of subordination
relations as indicated by the labels in the tree. The labels should be interpreted
as denoting different descriptive aspects. They will be referred to as DEScriptor
TYPEs. In fig 1 we find the following DES_TYPEs: MORPHOLOGY, TOPOGRAPHY, TYPE and
PART.

A DES_TYPE and its associated DES_TYPE_MANIFESTATION is called a DESCRIPTOR.

figure 1

'Medial collumfraktur, som är inkilad.'[1])

       (MORPHOLOGY (*FRAKTUR (TOPOGRAPHY (*COLLUM (PART *MEDIAL)))
                     (TYPE *INKILAD)))

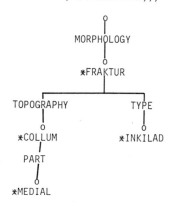

[1]) 'Medial collum fracture which is impacted.'

In a simple descriptor the manifestation consists of a CONCEPTUAL WORD, e g *ME-DIAL, *COLLUM, *FRAKTUR. (PART *MEDIAL) is an example of a simple descriptor.

In a complex descriptor the manifestation is itself a descriptor or a DESCRIPTION. A description is a conceptual word followed by any number of associated descriptors (simple or complex). (*COLLUM (PART *MEDIAL)) is an example of a description. It appears as the descriptor type manifestation of the complex descriptor (TOPOGRAPHY (*COLLUM (PART *MEDIAL))).

The semantic representation of a sentence is a descriptor.

Processing a complete report, the descriptors resulting from the analysis of the individual sentences should be associated to form a descriptor, representing the report as a whole. I will base this association process on the following text linguistic assumptions about a report.

The first sentence of a report, and, more specific, the head of its subject NP, as defined by the rules in our grammar, introduces the object to be described, the head object. Each following sentence contributes to the specification of the head object from a new aspect, presenting a new descriptor to be included in its description. For the sake of illustration, let us look at fig 2.

The first sentence of the report, being a paraphrase of 'Medial collumfraktur i vänster höftled.' introduces 'fraktur' as the head object of the report. The analysis of this sentence also gives a description of 'fraktur', with the descriptors (TOPOGRAPHY ...) and (REGION ...).

The recognition of (CAUSE ...) and (DISPLACEMENT ...) as descriptors of 'fraktur' is based on the text linguistic assumptions.

The use of the relative clause in the sentence 'Medial collumfraktur, som är inkilad.' enforces the explicit stating of the head object once again.

figure 2

'Vänster höftled: Medial collumfraktur. O-fall 720314. Medial collumfraktur,
som är inkilad. Ingen nämnvärd felställning.' 2)

```
    (MORPHOLOGY (*FRAKTUR (TOPOGRAPHY (*COLLUM (PART *MEDIAL)))
                         (REGION (*HÖFT (SIDE *VÄ)))
                         (CAUSE (*OFALL (DATE *720314)))
                         (TYPE *INKILAD)
                         (DISPLACEMENT (QUANTITY *INGEN_NÄMNVÄRD))))
```

2) 'Left hip joint: Medial collum fracture. Accident 720314. Medial collum
    fracture which is impacted. No displacement worth mentioning.'

Consequently, the process of incorporating a sentence descriptor into a report
descriptor must include a first step of pattern matching, where an attempt is
made to match the individual sentence descriptor with the report descriptor in
order to avoid a repetition of information. If there is a match, this step also
gives the correct place of insertion of the new piece of information, overriding
the text structure rules.

AN OUTLINE OF THE KNOWLEDGE ACQUISITION PROCESS

When we start analyzing the first report, the system has an embryo of a knowledge
base at its disposal, consisting of a dictionary, a grammar and some text linguistic rules. These three components define the context, the situation, so far. In
the dictionary we store functional words (prepositions, conjunctions etc) and
conceptual words (fracture, hip, inkilad etc). The conceptual words are marked
according to the descriptor type of which they are a manifestation. The grammar
covers the grammatical constructions which we expect to meet. It also relates the
grammatical constituents to their corresponding descriptors by means of semantic
rules. In that sense the system is complete, were it not for the exceptions to the
text structure rules and the grammatical ambiguities.

As a result of the processing of the first report we will get a report descriptor
which should be stored together with the formatted information about the same report, e g patient identification. It should also contribute to the system's general knowledge about the subject matter. This knowledge contribution should take
the shape of adding new pieces of information to the conceptual words. These
pieces of information should be identical to the descriptor types, appearing in
the descriptions of the same conceptual words in the report descriptor. Looking
back at fig 2 we state that *FRAKTUR will be supplied with the descriptor type
list (TOPOGRAPHY REGION CAUSE TYPE DISPLACEMENT), *COLLUM with the list (PART)
etc.

In the process of augmenting the descriptor type list of a certain conceptual
word, we must make sure that a descriptor type intended for insertion is not
already present. We must also be careful that there is no conflict between the
information already present and the additions we propose. If such a conflict
would be detected, we must have a means for solving it. It is an indication of
an uncorrect analysis. I intend to solve such conflicts, relying on the varying
strength in different grammatical relations, on grammatical valence criteria.

As a starting point for the differentiation between the relations we state that
the grammatical relations between the words within a sentence are more reliable
than the relations between the sentences, i e the rules in the grammar are prior
to the text structure rules. The relation between an attribute and its adjacent
noun is prior to the relation between a noun and a following prepositional phrase

etc. Consequently, in building the descriptor type lists we must include a stating of the origin of the relations. Detection of a conflict between the information already present and the new information means restructuring either the old or the new information, depending on its reliability in terms of grammatical valence criteria.

THE PARSER

The approach I have taken makes high demands on the parser. Here I have chosen to work within the framework suggested by Kay (see ref) and have made an INTERLISP implementation of his chart-analysis strategy. Fig 3 gives an overview over the main components of CHARTANALYS for this application.

figure 3

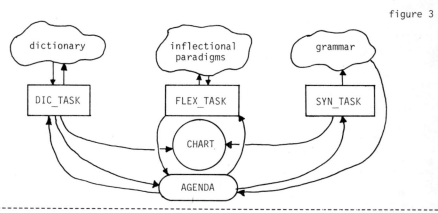

The dictionary, the inflectional paradigms and the grammar represent the application- and language-specific information. The CHART represents the sentence with its associated information in its varying shapes during the processing. The AGENDA handles the 'book-keeping' of the tasks to be carried out during the parsing procedure. DIC_TASK, FLEX_TASK and SYN_TASK are modules which take care of the dictionary look-up procedure, reference to the inflectional paradigms and reference to the grammar. In other words, they expand a dictionary task, an inflectional task and a syntactical task, respectively. All the actions during the parsing are formulated as tasks, being administrated by the agenda.

A nice consequence of this strategy is that we can follow each step of the analysis by the tasks, a fact of vital importance in building and testing the grammar. We can choose to have all the different types of tasks displayed or only one or two types. These choices are given as options to the top level function SYNT_ ANALYS. If we want to study the dictionary look-up and the inflectional analysis procedures, only, we can use the function MORF_ANALYS which as input takes an isolated word form and options as to whether we want both the dictionary tasks and the inflectional tasks displayed. Optionally, we can also display the final chart.

The dictionary keys are organized as a kind of binary letter tree, where common initial strings are represented only once. For the sake of illustration, imagine we have the following dictionary keys: HÖ (short for HÖGER), HÖFT, HÖGER, I, MED and MEDIAL. Given as an alphabetically sorted list to the function BUILD_DIC, they will be converted into a tree, as displayed in fig 4.

figure 4

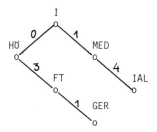

Let us study how searching in this tree is carried out in CHARTANALYS, following the example (MORF_ANALYS 'MEDIALA).

The processing starts by building a chart, representing the word form 'MEDIALA:

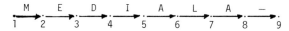

The chart consists of VERTICES (1 to 9), connected by directed, labelled EDGEs (1 - 2 M, 2 - 3 E, etc). In an initial chart there is always only one edge connecting two vertices. (For purely technical reasons MORF_ANALYS adds the end mark '_'.)

Then the first task of the agenda is activated - a dictionary task operating on the first edge of the chart, trying to match its label with the first letter of the first node in the dictionary, i e M - I. There is no match and a new task is created for the same edge and the following dictionary node. Since I precedes M in the alphabetic order, we are supposed to follow an arc in the dictionary tree labelled 1 to find the following node. Our new task will amount to a comparison between M and the first letter of the node MED. This task gives a match, and a new task is created for the next edge and the next letter of the same dictionary node (E - E). As a result of this match we will have the new task (D - D). This match is different from the previous ones, since it also means that we have found a complete dictionary key, i e MED. A reference to the dictionary information, associated with this key, however, shows that it represents a full word form, a preposition, and, consequently, it can't be our candidate. The input word and the key MED differ in the 4th position (I - blank), a fact which takes us to the node IAL by the dictionary arc labelled 4. In subsequent dictionary tasks (I - I, A - A, L - L) we find a new dictionary key candidate, i e MEDIAL. Its associated dictionary information tells us that it represents a stem, and it also gives a reference to the corresponding inflectional paradigm.

Fig 5 shows the dictionary information, associated with the key MEDIAL.

figure 5

```
(MEDIAL ((STEM (((SEM *MEDIAL)
                 (CLASS MOD)
                 (FLEX F4)
                 (FORM (12)))))))
```

The general structure of the dictionary information accounts for a great variety of homographs to be represented, e g homography between a stem and a word form, between two stems, belonging to the same grammatical category (or to different grammatical categories), between two forms of the same lexeme etc. SEM gives the

reference to the atom *MEDIAL which carries the descriptor type information. The
form information (FORM (12)) applies to the zero-ending, 12 being the index to
the corresponding element of the form value array.

The inflectional paradigms are organized in the same way as the dictionary keys
and the search follows the same principles. Back to our example. A new task, an
inflectional task, is initiated, operating on the edge (7 - 8 A) and the first
node of the paradigm tree. After a number of tasks we will find the appropriate
suffix with its information and we are ready to draw a new edge in the chart, from
the first to the last vertex, labelled with the total information from the dictionary entry and from the suffix:

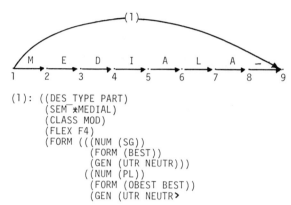

```
(1): ((DES_TYPE PART)
      (SEM *MEDIAL)
      (CLASS MOD)
      (FLEX F4)
      (FORM (((NUM (SG))
              (FORM (BEST))
              (GEN (UTR NEUTR)))
             ((NUM (PL))
              (FORM (OBEST BEST))
              (GEN (UTR NEUTR>
```

SYNT_ANALYS takes as its input the full sentence and the optional parameters. Its
output is the sentence descriptor, being identical to the label of the edge from
the first to the last vertex of the chart.

Fig 6 presents the final chart of the sentence 'Medial collumfraktur, som är inkilad.'

figure 6

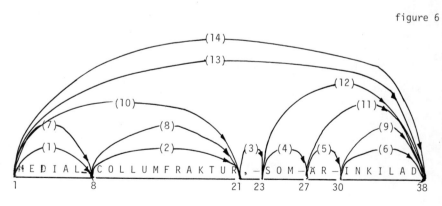

```
(14): G1  (MORPH (*FRAKTUR (TOP (*COLLUM (PART *MEDIAL)))
                           (TYPE *INKILAD)))
```

figure 6
cont

(13): G2 (NP (<DESCRIP (MORPH (*FRAKTUR (TOP (*COLLUM (PART *MEDIAL)))
                                          (TYPE *INKILAD
            (FORM (((NUM (SG))
                    (FORM (OBEST))
                    (GEN UTR>

(12): G6 (REL_CLAUSE ((DESCRIP (TYPE *INKILAD))
                      (FORM (((NUM (SG))
                              (FORM (OBEST))
                              (GEN UTR>

(11): G7 (VP ((DESCRIP (TYPE *INKILAD))
              (FORM (((NUM (SG))
                      (FORM (OBEST))
                      (GEN UTR>

(10): G4 (NP (<DESCRIP (MORPH (*FRAKTUR (TOP (*COLLUM (PART *MEDIAL>
              (FORM (((GEN UTR)
                      (CASE (NOM))
                      (NUM (SG))
                      (FORM (OBEST>

 (9): G5 (MOD_PH ((DESCRIP (TYPE *INKILAD))
                  (FORM (((NUM (SG PL))
                          (CASE (NOM))
                          (GEN (UTR NEUTR>

 (8): G3 (NP (<DESCRIP (MORPH (*FRAKTUR (TOP *COLLUM>
              <FORM (((GEN (UTR))
                      (CASE (NOM))
                      (NUM (SG))
                      (FORM (OBEST>
              (COMP T>

 (7): G5 (MOD_PH ((DESCRIP (PART *MEDIAL))
                  (FORM (((NUM (SG))
                          (FORM (OBEST))
                          (GEN (UTR>

 (6): L2 ((DES_TYPE TYPE)
          (SEM *INKILAD)
          (CLASS MOD)
          (FORM (((NUM (SG))
                  (FORM (OBEST))
                  (GEN (UTR>

 (5): L3 ((CLASS AUX)
          (FORM (((TEMP (PRES>

 (4): L4 ((CLASS REL)
          (FORM (((NUM (SG PL))
                  (CASE (NOM))
                  (GEN (UTR NEUTR>

 (3): L5 ((CLASS COMMA))

figure 6
cont

```
(2): L1 (<DESCRIP (MORPH (*FRAKTUR (TOP *COLLUM>
                          (SEM *COLLUMFRAKTUR)
                          (CLASS N)
                          (GEN (UTR))
                          (FLEX F1)
                          (FORM (((GEN (UTR))
                                   (CASE (NOM))
                                  (NUM (SG))
                                  (FORM (OBEST>

(1): L2 ((DES_TYPE PART)
          (SEM *MEDIAL)
          (CLASS MOD)
          (FLEX F4)
          (FORM (((NUM (SG))
                  (FORM (OBEST))
                 (GEN (UTR>
```

The chart in fig 6 is a result of the application of the grammatical rules
G1 - G7 and of the lexical rules L1 - L5:

G1   S ⟶ NP   (S5)

G2   NP ⟶ NP COMMA REL_CLAUSE   (S2)

G3   NP ⟶ N   (S1)

G4   NP ⟶ MOD_PH NP   (S3)

G5   MOD_PH ⟶ MOD   (S1)

G6   REL_CLAUSE ⟶ REL VP   (S4)

G7   VP ⟶ AUX MOD_PH   (S4)

...

L1   N ⟶ collumfraktur, ...

L2   MOD ⟶ medial, inkilad, ...

L3   AUX ⟶ är, ...

L4   REL ⟶ som, ...

L5   COMMA ⟶ ','

...

Corresponding to the grammatical rules there are semantic rules. The semantic
rules account for the building of the descriptors. (The descriptors are included
in the label information.) In our example in fig 6, the semantic rules S1 - S5
have been activated.

S1 corresponds to the grammatical rules G3 and G5. It builds a simple descriptor,
consisting of the DES_TYPE and the SEM information from the dictionary entry of
the noun or modifier in question. The descriptors (PART *MEDIAL), (TYPE *INKILAD)

and (MORPH (*FRAKTUR (TOP *COLLUM))) in our example result from the application
of S1. The last descriptor needs a comment. 'Collumfraktur' is a compound and the
information about the relation between its components is given as a descriptor in
the dictionary. (Usually, the dictionary gives only the descriptor type information.)

S2 and S3 correspond to the grammatical rules G2 and G4, respectively. They both
operate by means of the function HEAD_MOD with the parameters HEAD and MOD.
Calling HEAD_MOD for G2 and G4 looks like (HEAD_MOD NP REL_CLAUSE) and
(HEAD_MOD NP MOD_PH), respectively. In these function calls NP, REL_CLAUSE and
MOD_PH are represented by their corresponding descriptors. HEAD_MOD accounts for
subordination between two descriptors.

S4 corresponds to G6 and G7. It selects as descriptor of the left-hand side
constituent of the grammatical rule the descriptor of the second component of
the right-hand side of the rule, i e of VP and MOD_PH, respectively. REL and AUX
don't add to the descriptors. They are functional words which have played their
role in the recognition of the syntactic constituents.

S5, finally, corresponds to G1, assigning to S the descriptor of NP.

The grammar is implemented as an augmented transition network. The states in the
grammar consist of functions to be evaluated. The analysis works from top to
bottom. Pushing and recursion are accounted for. Changes in the grammar don't
influence the parser as such.

CONCLUSION

Before we can tell, how far we can get by the strategy outlined above, the knowledge acquisition process must be implemented and tested. For the next future
I will concentrate on problems concerning the detection of conflicts in the knowledge base and on the specification of the grammatical valence criteria.

Reference

M. Kay, Lecture notes from the 3rd International Summer School of Computational
    and Mathematical Linguistics, Pisa 1974.

Computational Linguistics in Medicine, Schneider/Sågvall Hein, eds.
North-Holland Publishing Company, (1977)

A RULE-BASED APPROACH TO THE GENERATION OF ADVICE
AND EXPLANATIONS IN CLINICAL MEDICINE

Edward H. Shortliffe
Department of Medicine
Massachusetts General Hospital
Boston, Massachusetts

The MYCIN system is a large computer program designed to help
physicians select antibiotics for patients with septicemia or
meningitis. Although the system's emphasis is on the selection
of appropriate therapy for critically ill patients, it also
necessarily assists with certain aspects of infectious disease
diagnosis. This paper provides a brief overview of the program,
describing in particular its scheme for the representation of
clinical knowledge and the ways in which this representation
facilitates both the generation of advice and the explanation
of decisions. The encoding of knowledge in production rules,
which are analyzed for advice generation by a goal-oriented rule
interpreter, also permits a simple but powerful approach to
natural language understanding. Despite its limitations, this
approach provides an effective explanation capability without
addressing many of the complex problems encountered in computational linguistics. The flow of information between a user
and the MYCIN system is compared to that which occurs when a
physician seeks the advice of a human infectious disease consultant.

1. INTRODUCTION

As medical knowledge has expanded in recent decades, it has become evident that
the individual practitioner can no longer hope to acquire enough expertise to man-
age adequately the full range of clinical problems that will be encountered in his
practice. The general practitioner has accordingly become rare, and today's primary care physicians are beginning to graduate from family practice residencies
which recognize that "family doctoring" is a subspecialty in itself. Thus when a
patient's problem clearly falls outside the area of the attending physician's
expertise, consultations from experts in other subspecialties have become a well-
accepted part of medical practice. Such consultations are acceptable to doctors
in part because they maintain the primary physician's role as ultimate decision
maker. The consultation generally involves a dialog between the two physicians,
with the expert explaining the basis for his advice and the nonexpert seeking jus-

The MYCIN Project is located at Stanford University School of Medicine and is
supported by BHSRE Grant No. HS01544. Much of the work described in this report
was undertaken by other project members, notably A.C. Scott and W.J. Clancey, who
have devoted much of their time to improvements in the general question-answerer,
and R. Davis, who did most of the work on the reasoning status checker and on
knowledge acquisition capabilities. Other researchers involved with the work
have included J.S. Aikins, B.G. Buchanan, L.M. Fagan, and W.J. van Melle (computer
scientists), V.L. Yu, S.G. Axline, and S.N. Cohen (physicians), and S.M. Wraith
(clinical pharmacist). The research described has been undertaken on the SUMEX
computing facility, also located at Stanford University, and supported by BRB/NIH
Grant RR-00785.

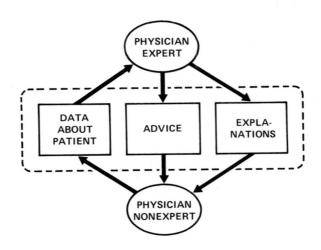

FIGURE 1 - Diagram summarizing the flow of information between
          physician and expert in the human consultation process.

tification of points he finds puzzling or questionable. A consultant who offered
dogmatic advice he was unwilling to discuss or defend would find his opinions
were seldom sought.

Fig. 1 shows a schematic view of the consultation process. The physician nonexpert gives information about his patient to the expert in response to questions
and, in return, receives advice and explanations. Thus there are actually three
kinds of information flow between the physician and his consultant. This paper
describes a computer program, termed MYCIN, which models the consultative process
by attending to all three kinds of information. It is our conviction that programs which ignore the explanation pathway will fail to be accepted by physicians
because they will see in such systems too severe a departure from the human consultation process (in which the primary physician is provided with sufficient
information to allow him to decide whether to follow the offered advice).

MYCIN is a LISP program designed to serve as a clinical consultant on the subject
of therapy selection for patients with infections. The program may be envisioned
as interposed between the expert and **nonexpert** in much the way that the large box
is positioned in Fig. 1. The difference is that the human expert can offer only
general knowledge to the program, not patient-specific decisions. The program
thus becomes the decision maker, using general medical knowledge from experts to
assess a specific patient and to give advice plus explanations for its judgments.

Fig. 2 details the organization of MYCIN relative to the human consultation process depicted in Fig. 1. As before, the nonexpert offers data about his patient
and in return receives both advice and, when desired, information via one of two
internal explanation mechanisms (the "General Question-Answerer"or the "Reasoning
Status Checker"). The basis for all decisions is domain-specific knowledge acquired from experts ("Static Knowledge"). A group of computer programs (the
"Rule Interpreter") uses this knowledge, and data about the specific patient, to

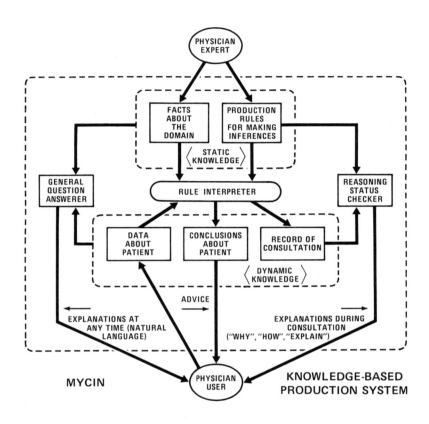

FIGURE 2 — Diagram summarizing the organization and flow of
information within MYCIN. The correlation between
this design and the human consultation process depicted in Fig. 1 is discussed in the text.

generate conclusions and, in turn, therapeutic advice. It simultaneously keeps a
record of what has happened, and this record is available to the explanation routines if the physician asks for justification or clarification of some conclusion
the program has reached. In the remainder of this paper some details of each of
these system components will be presented. More extensive discussions of this
material are also available [1-4].

2. KNOWLEDGE REPRESENTATION

2.1 Static Knowledge
Static knowledge refers to all data that are constant in the program and un-
changing from one consultation to the next.

2.1.1 Facts About The Domain
Much of the knowledge MYCIN requires is simple
statements of fact about the domain. These can generally be represented as
attribute-object-value triples, or as predicate statements. For example:

	(GRAMSTAIN E.COLI GRAMNEG)	i.e., the gramstain of e.coli is gram negative
or:	(STERILESITE BLOOD T)	i.e., the **blood** is normally sterile
or:	(STERILESITE MOUTH NIL)	i.e., the mouth is not normally sterile

2.1.2 Production Rules
In addition to simple facts, MYCIN requires judgmental
knowledge acquired from experts and available for use in analyzing a new patient.
Judgmental knowledge in MYCIN is expressed as production rules [5] which define
certain preconditions (the PREMISE) that allow a conclusion to be reached (the
ACTION) with a specified degree of confidence (the "certainty factor" [6]).
Although such rules are stored as LISP list structures, a series of routines is
available for translating them into English. For example:

> PREMISE: If the stain of the organism is gramneg, and
> the morphology of the organism is rod, and
> the aerobicity of the organism is anaerobic,
> ACTION: Then there is suggestive evidence (.7) that the
> identity of the organism is bacteroides.

Note that the _purpose_ of this rule is determination of organism identity. Rules
are classified and accessed in accordance with their purpose as described below.

2.2 Dynamic Knowledge
Dynamic knowledge refers to all data that are variable and change from one run of
the program to the next.

2.2.1 Data About The Patient - Acquired From The User
MYCIN asks questions of
the user, driven by a reasoning algorithm described below. These questions
generally ask the user to fill in the "value" in an attribute-object-value triple
(eg., "What is the patient's name?"), or to give the truth value of a predicate
(eg., "Is the patient a compromised host?"). Thus these data may be represented,
once acquired, in precisely the way that facts about the domain are represented
in the static knowledge base (see 2.1.1).

2.2.2 Data About The Patient - Generated By The Program
When the preconditions
in the PREMISE of a rule are found to hold, MYCIN executes the ACTION portion of
the rule and generates a new "fact" which can, once again, be represented as an
attribute-object-value triple. As discussed in 2.1.2, conclusions may also have
a confidence value associated with them, thereby requiring that the triple be
expanded to a quadruple:

> (IDENTITY ORGANISM-1 BACTEROIDES .7)   i.e., the identity of ORGANISM-1
> is bacteroides, with cer-
> tainty factor of .7

Predicates may be similarly expanded. Furthermore, by generalizing this scheme
to include representation of data acquired from the user, the physician may be
asked to express his confidence in the answer he gives when MYCIN asks a question.

2.2.3 Maintenance Of A Record Of The Consultation
A history of the consulta-

tion is the third variety of dynamic knowledge. The details of representation
need not be described here, but these data include records of which rules succeeded, which rules were tried but failed, how specific decisions were made, how
information was used, and why questions were asked.

3. THE PRODUCTION SYSTEM

3.1 The Rule Interpreter
This series of routines analyzes rules in the static knowledge base, determines
whether they apply to the patient under consideration, and if so draws the conclusions delineated in the ACTION portions of the rules. This process would
quickly become unmanageable as system knowledge grew if there were not a mechanism for selecting only the most relevant rules for a given patient. This is
accomplished by a goal-oriented approach described in detail elsewhere [1,7].
Briefly, as the rule interpreter examines the PREMISE of a rule, it notes whether
the relevant data needed to determine the truth of each precondition are already
known. If not, it digresses to examine those rules which make conclusions about
the data needed by the first rule. The PREMISE conditions of those rules may, in
turn, invoke additional rules, and in this way a reasoning network relevant to
the first rule is formed. As described in 2.1.2, since rules are classified according to their purpose, it is easy to identify all rules which may aid in determining the truth of a specific precondition. The entire process is initiated
by invoking a specific "Goal Rule" which defines MYCIN's task and is the only rule
necessarily invoked for every consultation. When MYCIN can find no rules for determining the truth of a precondition, it asks the user for the relevant data.
If the physician does not know the information either, the invoking rule is simply ignored.

3.2 Maintenance Of Initiative In The Hands Of The Physician
As was discussed above, a physician is not likely to accept a system such as
MYCIN if the program simply asks a series of questions and then presents a piece
of dogmatic advice as it terminates execution. The production system has therefore been provided with a series of "interrupts" that allow the physician to
digress with questions of his own or to demand justification for the line of
questioning on which MYCIN has embarked during the consultation. Whenever the
program asks a question, the user can temporarily refuse to answer and instead
call on the explanation capabilities described in the next section.

4. EXPLANATIONS

4.1 The Reasoning Status Checker (RSC)
This component of the explanation system deals with most questions that arise
during the consultation itself. Because the context of current reasoning about
the patient is well-defined, the physician can be given a great deal of information on the basis of a few simple commands that do not require natural language
processing. These commands are briefly described below; more extensive details
of their implementation are also available [3,4,7]. As shown in Fig. 2, the
reasoning status checker (RSC) uses only the knowledge base of rules and the current record of the consultation; the general question-answerer described in 4.2,
on the other hand, has access to all static and dynamic knowledge.

4.1.1 The WHY Command
Whenever MYCIN asks a question, the physician may prefer
not to answer initially and instead to inquire about the reasoning underlying the
questioning. Thus he may simply respond with the command WHY (i.e., "Why do you
think the information you are requesting may be useful?"). Since all questions
MYCIN asks are generated by rules, and since the rules are selected according to
their purpose as discussed in 3.1, an English translation of the rule under consideration generally serves as an adequate response to the WHY query. The RSC

therefor responds by displaying the current rule. In addition, it places an identifying number before each of the preconditions in the PREMISE and indicates
whether the condition is (a) already known to be true, or (b) still under investigation (note that one of the latter group of preconditions will have generated
MYCIN's current question to the user). The physician can in turn inquire why the
displayed rule was selected by asking WHY a second time, and the RSC will accordingly display the next rule in the reasoning network (see 3.1).

An experienced user will learn to seek higher level explanations by entering WHY
followed by a modifying number. The number tells the RSC the **relative size of the**
reasoning leap (roughly the number of chained rules) to compile into a single
explanation. If the physician finds the leap is in fact too large, the command
EXPLAIN provides a breakdown of the component reasoning steps.

4.1.2 <u>The HOW Command</u>   As discussed in the preceding section, when MYCIN displays a rule in response to the WHY command, it labels each precondition in the
PREMISE with a unique number. The physician may then respond to the displayed
explanation by entering HOW followed by one of the identifying labels. If the
reference condition is one that MYCIN has already concluded to be true, the RSC
assumes that the physician is asking "HOW did you decide that the specified precondition is true?" and answers by citing the relevant rules that it used to make
the decision. If, on the other hand, the cited condition has not yet been fully
investigated, MYCIN assumes the physician is asking "HOW will you decide if the
specified precondition is true?" and responds by citing the rules it intends to
try, only some of which may actually succeed.

4.2 <u>The General Question-Answerer (GQA)</u>
The general question-answerer (GQA) is a more comprehensive explanation system
which, at any time during or after the consultation session, has full access to
all static and dynamic knowledge in MYCIN (Fig. 2). Since it cannot make simple
assumptions based on context, as the RSC can do, and since it is important to
keep the system useable by a novice, the GQA must accept and answer questions expressed in natural language. MYCIN's rule-based knowledge representation scheme,
and some techniques borrowed from early work in computational linguistics [8-10],
permit a straightforward but powerful approach to interpreting simple English
questions without contending with several of the complex problems of natural
language understanding. The details of this approach have been described elsewhere [4,11].

4.2.1 <u>Questions About Static Knowledge</u>   The ability to retrieve information
from the static knowledge base gives the GQA a tutorial capability. Since the
static knowledge is acquired from experts, the GQA can essentially act as an intermediary between an expert and a physician seeking general information about
the infectious disease field. The user might ask simple questions of fact (eg.,
"Which culture sites are normally considered sterile?") or questions regarding
judgments stored in rules. Questions of the second variety are called "rule-
retrieval" questions because they may be answered simply by identifying and displaying English versions of relevant rules from the knowledge base. Retrieval
may be keyed to the rule PREMISE (eg., "How do you use the gram stain of an organism?"), the ACTION (eg., "When do you decide an organism might be a streptococcus?"), or to both the PREMISE and ACTION (eg., "Do you ever use the morphology
of an organism to determine its identity?"). Furthermore, a question may deal
with a specific rule (eg., "What is rule037?"). Note that none of these questions
refers to a specific consultation and thus requires no access to the dynamic
knowledge base (Fig. 2).

4.2.2 <u>Questions About Dynamic Knowledge</u>   Although the RSC permits inquiries
regarding the dynamic knowledge base, its scope is limited by the context of the
current question being asked by MYCIN (see 4.1). If the physician wishes to ask
more general questions regarding the status of MYCIN's reasoning, or if he wishes

to review the program's decisions after the consultation is complete and MYCIN is
no longer questioning him, the GQA gives him free access to all information about
the specific consultation. Once again, the user might ask simple questions of
fact (eg., "From what site was CULTURE-2 obtained?") or questions regarding the
basis for MYCIN's judgments. The second variety is again a "rule-retrieval" question, but is keyed to the consultation record in dynamic data rather than to the
knowledge base of rules in static data. Thus questions may again reference the
PREMISE (eg., "How did you use the gram stain of ORGANISM-1?"), the ACTION (eg.,
"What makes you think ORGANISM-2 might be a streptococcus?"), or both (eg., "Did
you use the morphology of ORGANISM-1 to determine its identity?"). Note that
these questions parallel the examples in 4.2.1 but that they are consultation-
specific and thus request the retrieval not of <u>all</u> relevant rules, but only those
that were actually used successfully in the specified context. Finally, one may
again wish to ask about a specific rule (eg., "Did you use rule037 when considering ORGANISM-1?").

5. KNOWLEDGE ACQUSITION

The only component of Fig. 2 not yet discussed is the crucial step of acquiring
domain-specific knowledge from experts and coding it for storage in the static
knowledge base. When MYCIN was first being developed, such knowledge was acquired by extensive meetings during which infectious disease experts and computer
scientists discussed specific patients and attempted to analyze and extract the
individual facts and rules they were utilizing. Recently extensive work has been
devoted to the problem of automating the knowledge acquisition process in sessions
involving clinical experts interacting with MYCIN directly. This problem has
been thoroughly explored in another publication [3] and will not be discussed
further here.

6. CONCLUSIONS

A rule-based expert system is described which uses artificial intelligence techniques, and a model of the interaction between physicians and human consultants,
to attempt to satisfy the demands of a user community that is often reluctant
to experiment with computer technology. An ability to explain decisions, and
thus to respond to simple questions expressed in natural language, is emphasized.
The representation of expert knowledge in production rules facilitates greatly
the generation of explanations without requiring solutions to several of the complex problems encountered in computational linguistics.

References

[1] Shortliffe, E.H. <u>Computer-Based Medical Consultations: MYCIN</u>. Elsevier/
    North Holland, New York, 1976.

[2] Davis, R., Buchanan, B.G., and Shortliffe, E.H. Production rules as an ap-
    proach to knowledge-based consultation systems. <u>Artificial Intelligence 8</u>,
    15-45 (1977).

[3] Davis, R. <u>Applications Of Meta Level Knowledge To The Construction, Main-
    tenance, And Use Of Large Knowledge Bases</u>. Doctoral dissertation, Stanford
    University, June 1976. Also available as AIM-283, Stanford Artificial In-
    telligence Laboratory, Stanford University, July 1976.

[4] Scott, A.C., Clancey, W.J., Davis, R., and Shortliffe, E.H. Explanation
    capabilities of knowledge-based production systems. <u>Amer. J. Computational</u>

Linguistics, Microfiche 62, 1977. Also available as TR HPP-77-1, Heuristic
Programming Project, Stanford University, March 1977.

[5] Davis, R., and King, J. An overview of production systems. To appear in
Machine Representations of Knowledge (Machine Intelligence 8, eds. E.W. El-
cock and D. Michie), John Wylie, New York, 1976. Also available as AIM-271,
Stanford Artificial Intelligence Laboratory, Stanford University, October
1975.

[6] Shortliffe, E.H., and Buchanan, B.G. A model of inexact reasoning in medicine
Math. Biosci. 23,351-379 (1975).

[7] Shortliffe, E.H., Davis, R., Buchanan, B.G., Axline, S.G., Green, C.C., and
Cohen, S.N. Computer-based consultations in clinical therapeutics: explana-
tion and rule-acquisition capabilities of the MYCIN system. Comput. Biomed.
Res. 8,303-320 (1975).

[8] Green, B.F., Wolf, A.K., Chomsky, C., and Laughery, K. BASEBALL: an automatic question-answerer (1961). In Computers and Thought (E.A. Feigenbaum
and J. Feldman, eds.), pp.207-216, McGraw Hill, San Francisco, 1963.

[9] Colby, K., Weber, S., and Hilf, F. Artificial paranoia. Artificial Intelligence 2,1-25 (1971).

[10] Quillian, M.R. Semantic memory. In Semantic Information Processing (M.
Minsky, ed.), pp.227-270, MIT Press, Cambridge, MA. (1968).

[11] Shortliffe, E.H. MYCIN: A Rule-Based Computer Program For Advising Physi-
cians Regarding Antimicrobial Therapy Selection. Doctoral dissertation,
Stanford University, October 1974. Also available as AIM-251, Stanford
Artificial Intelligence Laboratory, Stanford University, November 1974.

Computational Linguistics in Medicine, Schneider/Sågvall Hein, eds.
North-Holland Publishing Company, (1977)

ANALYZING AND SIMULATING
TAKING THE HISTORY OF THE PRESENT ILLNESS:
CONTEXT FORMATION

Stephen G. Pauker, M.D., and Peter Szolovits, Ph.D.[*]

Clinical Decision Making Group
Department of Medicine
New England Medical Center Hospital
Tufts University School of Medicine
Boston, Massachusetts, USA
and
Laboratory for Computer Science
Massachusetts Institute of Technology
Cambridge, Massachusetts, USA

The history of the present illness is the cornerstone of the
physician's diagnostic process, and the acquisition of that
history is basically a problem in context formation, hypothesis
generation and hypothesis evaluation. The problem domain facing
the physician taking this history is quite broad and must be
narrowed sharply to allow efficient pursuit of hypotheses about
the patient's disease process. This problem of context formation
is shared by the field of computational linguistics and many of
the disciplines of artificial intelligence. This report describes
our research in the modeling of this diagnostic process in a
computer laboratory. Our methodology consisted of protocol analysis
and subsequent theory formation about the physician's cognitive
processes. These theories were implemented in a computer program
which was then iteratively tested and improved by comparing its
behavior in dealing with actual cases to that of experienced
clinicians presented with identical cases. This program dealt with
the isolated diagnostic phase of physician performance. Ultimately,
this history-taking process must be driven by downstream
consequences, i.e., the costs and benefits of testing and treatment,
and any history-taking program must be carefully interfaced with
other programs that deal with therapeutic decision making.

The physician is primarily a problem-solver: faced with a patient who
presents with a set of complaints, the physician must synthesize the situation
into a set of reasonable hypotheses and must then formulate a plan for further
diagnostic work-up and for eventual treatment. In many cases the patient could
be suffering from any of a large set of diseases involving many different organ
systems. The development of reasonable and coherent hypotheses from the patient's
"chief complaint" and from the data acquired during the physician-patient
encounter is a process which is broadly termed "taking the history of the present
illness." That process is initially one of context formation. Before making any
decisions about diagnostic tests or treatments, or indeed before asking more than
the most cursory, automatic, descriptive questions, the physician must limit his

---
[*]Drs. William B. Schwartz, Jerome P. Kassirer and G. Anthony Gorry were major
contributors to the work described in this report. This research was supported
in part by the Health Resources Administration, US Public Health Service, under
Grant 1R01MB00107-01 from the Bureau of Health Manpower and under Grant 00911-01
from the National Center for Health Services Research.
Address reprint requests to Dr. Stephen Pauker, New England Medical Center
Hospital, 171 Harrison Avenue, Boston, Massachusetts, USA 02111

domain of consideration to an appropriately narrow context. It is this process of context formation which we shall address in this paper.

This conference on computational linguistics in medicine is an appropriate forum for discussion of this research for several reasons. First, the problems of context formation, hypothesis generation, and hypothesis evaluation are faced by researchers in computational linguistics, both on the level of resolving references and on the level of semantics. Indeed, many of the tools being developed in natural language laboratories are now finding application in medical diagnosis, including languages like MACLISP[3], OWL[8], and CONNIVER[7]. Second, the problem domain of medicine is sufficiently well constrained and contains a rich enough vocabulary to form a fruitful working world for basic research in linguistics and artificial intelligence. Third, the domain of medical diagnosis provides recognizable, expert problem solvers -- experienced clinicians.

Our methodology has been to observe the problem-solving behavior of these experienced physicians and then to formulate theories about their behavior. These theories are expressed as computer programs and are then tested in a computer laboratory by "presenting" the programs with a series of actual cases. The problem-solving behaviors of these programs are then contrasted to those of a panel of clinicians presented with similar cases. Discrepancies between the program's and the physician's behavior are then analyzed in detail. These analyses provide insight into the inadequacies of our evolving theories of clinical cognition. Those theories are then expanded, modified, and incorporated into revised programs. This iterative process has allowed us to formulate a theory of clinical cognition.

In this presentation we shall first elaborate our elementary theory of clinical cognition and shall describe the computer program which embodies it. We shall discuss the shortcomings of the program and contrast its behavior as a context former to that of other artificial intelligence programs that deal with medical diagnosis. Finally, we shall discuss the general limitations of numerical diagnostic algorithms and make some suggestions about the eventual solution to those limitations.

CLINICAL HYPOTHESIS FORMATION

The actual behavior of expert clinicians differs sharply from the approach to clinical problem solving taught in most medical schools. At present we often suggest that the student take a slow, methodical approach to diagnosis, considering every possible diagnosis in turn, and that he gradually exclude those diagnoses which do not explain the findings at hand. In contrast we have found that only medical students and inexperienced physicians use that approach. Expert clinicians utilize that diagnostic style only when faced with a case far afield from their area of expertise.

In contrast, an expert physician working within his domain of expertise seems to make an initial guess at the nature of the problem at hand -- often on the basis of what appears to be little information. This zero-order hypothesis then forms the basis for further data acquisition. As additional clinical information about the patient is gathered, it is evaluated with respect to the current working hypotheses. When a sufficient number of inconsistencies arise or when a critical finding cannot be explained, the expert then revises his working hypotheses. Since he has usually expended a moderate amount of intellectual effort in his development of the earlier hypotheses, he is sometimes reticent to make this switch and may go to some lengths in an attempt to find reasonable explanations for the inconsistencies.

This step of hypothesis switching is central to the nature of expertise. The true expert only rarely backs-up, unwinding his tangled web of hypotheses, and turns to a totally new hypothesis. Rather, his knowledge base contains a richly interconnected network of information which allows him to move laterally from one hypothesis to another, while maintaining many of the links and conclusions which he has already processed. For example, if he were considering nephrotic syndrome as his working hypothesis and he discovered that the neck veins were massively distended while the lung fields were relatively clear, he might move directly to consideration of constrictive pericarditis. In clinical parlance, this direct lateral motion is known as differential diagnosis and is a recognized skill of the expert consultant.

Of course, much more is involved in going from a chief complaint to a coherent plan for diagnosis and management. One must consider the sequence of information gathering (i.e., in what order should questions be asked and should tests be done?), termination criteria (i.e., when should the diagnostic phase be ended and the treatment selection phase be begun?), and how the choice of treatment should be made. This paper will not focus on those areas in depth. It suffices to say that we believe that all of these downstream choices must be based on the utilities, or relative values, of the various potential outcomes. Of course, the technique of decision analysis can be an effective approach to these problems, but to use that technique effectively, the diagnostic phase must provide outputs that can be mapped into probabilities, or relative likelihoods for the various diagnoses under consideration. For this reason it is important to develop diagnostic programs that can produce their measures of "goodness of fit" on a probability scale, rather than on an arbitrary one.

For the moment, let us return to the issue of the generation of the initial hypothesis by the clinician -- the step of context formation. We believe that this is the key step of the diagnostic process, since the expert's knowledge base will allow him to move efficiently from one hypothesis to the next, once the initial context has been established. Indeed, it is just the efficiency of this hypothesis or context switching which makes it reasonable for the expert to make an initial "wild" guess. If errors in that guess were to require the physician to unwind his web of conclusions to point zero, then making such a guess would be quite inefficient. If that were the case, the physician could only afford to jump into a narrow context if he were almost certain that his hypotheses were correct. Indeed, this describes the behavior of the medical student or the inexperienced clinician who spends a great deal of time in rather broad contexts which are only gradually narrowed. In contrast, the experienced clinician's expertise allows him to jump rapidly to a very narrow context (which is quite efficient for many of the information processing techniques which he utilizes), since his knowledge network will allow him to switch contexts at relatively low cost.

The process by which the clinician makes his initial guess is one that we have termed "triggering." When presented with certain key findings or triggers, he rapidly establishes a context for further exploration. For example, when told that a patient who has edema had a preceding pharyngitis, the clinician immediately hypothesizes that the patient has. acute post-streptococcal glomerulonephritis. Similarly, when a fifty year old man presents with exertional chest discomfort, the cardiologist will immediately jump into the context of angina pectoris which will have differential diagnostic pointers to aortic stenosis, hypertrophic cardiomyopathy and the like. When a context is triggered, an entire region of the physician's knowledge base appears to come into active consideration. Furthermore, other findings which would not ordinarily have been triggers themselves, e.g., headache, take on trigger status. In this example, once the context of acute glomerulonephritis has been activated, the finding of headache will trigger consideration of hypertensive encephalopathy, a complication of acute glomerulonephritis. Of course, the finding of headache might have already had trigger status for other contexts, e.g., brain tumor.

THE PRESENT ILLNESS PROGRAM

We shall now turn to a description of the program[4] which evolved in this research effort. This program was originally written in the CONNIVER[7] language, a superset of MACLISP[3]. It ran on a Digital Equipment Corporation PDP-10 computer. Since that time, the program has been partially re-written directly in MACLISP and is now much more efficient. The original version suffered from the problems inherent to a distributed control structure. The revised program uses a central control structure and uses a discrimination net to accomplish pattern matching. The domain of these programs is a patient who presents with the chief complaint of edema. Since our area of interest is the consultant's cognitive processes, we have not attempted to interact these programs directly with the patient. Rather, we have assumed that the primary physician will interact with the program much in the way he interacts with a consultant on the wards.

For clarity, let us divide the process of taking the history of the present illness into two intertwined components -- diagnosis and question selection. By diagnosis we mean the passive process of changing contexts and hypotheses in response to clinical information, as it is provided. A model for this process is the physician solving the puzzle of a clinical-pathologic conference, or CPC. That setting, found in most academic institutions, pits the clinician against the pathologist. The clinician is presented with only a written summary of the case from which he must deduce the proper diagnosis. The pathologist, who knows the correct diagnosis based on either the autopsy or a biopsy, then comments on the clinician's diagnoses. In such a forum, the clinician can specify neither the order nor the type of information provided. He can only react passively to the written summary of the case. In contrast, question selection is the active process of choosing which additional information to request and in what order tests should be performed. Although the expert consultant is more often faced with this latter situation, the passive diagnostic process certainly lies at the core of question selection. Which questions are asked and which tests are ordered will depend on the information which these additional data might provide in the context of the working hypotheses. These choices will also depend on the relative costs of additional data.

Components of the Program

The original present illness program consisted of three major components: 1) the supervisory program, 2) the short-term memory and 3) the long-term memory. These components interacted with the patient-specific data, and that interaction resulted in the system's behavior. The patient-specific data are a collection of facts about the patient provided by the physician-user either spontaneously or in response to specific questions. The supervisory program acts as the interface to the physician-user and modulates the interaction of the data that he provides with the short-term memory. The two memories are content-addressable. The long-term memory contains the system's knowledge base, while the short-term memory provides the battleground where competing patterns are matched against each new finding.

Operation of the Program

Data are acquired from the physician by the supervisory program, and after appropriate checks and modifications, those data are placed in the short-term memory. The short-term memory also contains a number of programs, called demons, which are compiled from the declarative knowledge of the long-term memory. Each demon has an associated pattern or key. When a patient-specific finding matches one of these keys, the associated program is "run" and various modifications are made in the short-term memory. These modifications may themselves cause other data to be placed in that memory, and these secondary data may cause other programs to run.

In this environment, let us first consider the role of the supervisory program. Before incoming data are exposed to the turbulent fury of the short-term memory, certain checks are made to minimize the amount of inappropriate activity which might ensue. First, it is important to assure that the incoming findings are specified as narrowly as possible. For example, the effect of (EDEMA FACIAL SYMMETRICAL PAINLESS) is to match a smaller set of patterns than would be matched by (EDEMA PRESENT). Second, it is often useful to provide additional data to "pave the way" for patient-specific findings that are quite general. For example, before placing (EDEMA PEDAL) in short-term memory, it is useful to explore the history for dyspnea, jaundice, renal disease, or varicose veins. Third, it is quite important to anticipate any inconsistencies which might arise in the incoming data.

At this moment, let us digress to consider the general issue of inconsistent data. Several types of inconsistencies can arise in the incoming patient-specific data stream. A finding may be internally inconsistent or may be inconsistent with the program's knowledge of physiology, e.g., a serum sodium concentration of 14 meq/liter. This type of inconsistency is usually discovered locally by the data entry routine and can be corrected by re-asking the question. Next, a finding can be inconsistent with other findings known about the case, e.g., red cell casts are inconsistent with the absence of at least microscopic hematuria. In these situations, heuristics are often available to advise the program which finding is more likely to be valid. In this example, microscopic hematuria is usually a reliable finding, while red cell casts are often confused with other material in the urinary sediment. In this case, the action which the program will take depends on the order that the findings were presented to the program. If the finding of red cell casts was presented after the finding of absent hematuria, the casts are neglected. If the order was reversed, then the finding of casts would have to be removed from the short-term memory and all consequences of that finding would need to be undone. Rather than do all the bookkeeping necessary to process such "backing up," we re-initialize the short-term memory and re-enter the correct findings, omitting the one to be neglected. This procedure occurs internally and is invisible to the user. Yet another type of inconsistency is a finding which contradicts conclusions already drawn by the program about the case. Since such conclusions were often drawn at considerable expense and since they often serve to explain other findings in the case, it is desirable to smooth over the inconsistency by finding a reasonable explanation for it. For example, if the program had already concluded that chronic hypertension was present (based on electrocardiographic and fundoscopic findings) and the physician were to state that the blood pressure is normal, then the program would seek to explain the absence of an elevated blood pressure by asking questions about antihypertensive therapy and intercurrent myocardial infarctions. We should note that this latter type of inconsistency will give rise to some asymmetry of the program's behavior. If the finding of a normal blood pressure were entered first, then the conclusion about the presence of chronic hypertension would be made with more reticence, whereas if that conclusion were reached first, then the program would go to some length to "explain" the normal blood pressure. Although such asymmetrical behavior might raise questions on a theoretical level, it corresponds quite well to the behavior of human problem-solvers.

Returning to the supervisory program, we recall that these various checks on the incoming data are performed before those data enter the short-term memory. These heuristic checks might result in the data being neglected or modified, might result in additional data being gathered and placed in short-term memory before this datum is placed there, or might result in modifications to the present contents of the short-term memory. Initially, the short-term memory contains only those demons that correspond to trigger findings. When a patient-specific finding matches the pattern of one of these demons, the associated program is run and causes hypotheses to be moved from the long-term memory to the short-term memory. The long-term memory consists of a network of interconnected frames[2], each of which is a chunk of data about a small subset of medical knowledge. Frames can describe diseases (e.g., acute glomerulonephritis), clinical states (e.g., nephrotic syndrome), or physiological states (e.g., sodium retention). Each frame consists of a set of findings which might be found in a prototypical example of the entity which the frame describes, sets of rules for both establishing and excluding the existence of that entity in a given case, a scoring function for measuring the fit of the frame to the case, and a set of pointers to other frames. These links are differential diagnosis links to frames often confused with the frame under consideration, links to clinical entities which often complicate the entity under consideration, and links to entities which could cause the entity under consideration. For example, the frame for acute glomerulonephritis is linked to the frames for vasculitis, sodium retention, and streptococcal infection.

When a finding matches a trigger in the short-term memory, the associated frame is brought from the long-term memory to the short-term memory, and consequently demons corresponding to all the frame's findings (not just the trigger findings) are allowed to run in the short-term memory. Other findings which are "closely" related to the activated frame (e.g., STREPTOCOCCAL-INFECTION which is linked to ACUTE-GLOMERULONEPHRITIS by a single "caused-by" link) are thereby brought nearer to the short-term memory where they too are allowed to run the demons associated with all their findings. These frames which are nearby the short-term memory are called "semi-active" and all of their findings take on the status of trigger findings, analogous to the hypertensive encephalopathy example presented earlier. If subsequent findings match these new demons, then the frames associated with them will be activated. These changes in the short-term memory form a new context for the diagnostic process.

Goodness of Fit

In the initial version of the program, the problem of pattern matching was handled by the CONNIVER data base, which was not designed for this complex pattern-matching task and which was consequently unacceptably slow. Our current version of the program uses a discrimination net for this task and runs several orders of magnitude faster. At this point, let us consider the pattern-matching task. Since findings may be incompletely specified, it can be difficult to know whether a finding matches a given key or pattern sufficiently well. For example, a pattern specifying (EDEMA (NOT PAINFUL)) should match (EDEMA PEDAL) and (EDEMA PAINLESS), but a pattern specifying (EDEMA PAINLESS) should not match (EDEMA PEDAL) since the character of PAINLESSness was not specified but was required by the latter pattern, whereas the pattern (EDEMA (NOT PAINFUL)) could match either PAINLESS or "pain status unknown."

At this point, let us consider the measures of the fit between the case and the hypothesis. A numerical score is used, and it consists of two components: 1) the fit of the case to the frame and 2) the ability of the frame to account for the findings of the case. In other words, there are two general types of frame-data mismatches. First, an expected finding may be absent, e.g., a patient thought to have constrictive pericarditis may not have inspiratory elevation of his neck veins (Kussmaul's sign). Second, an abnormal finding may not be explained by the frame, e.g., the patient may have hypoproteinemia which would not be explained by pericarditis. In this example, nephrotic syndrome might provide a better fit.

Since the long-term memory is organized into small chunks of knowledge, several frames must often be combined to form a coherent hypothesis. For example, typical acute post-streptococcal glomerulonephritis might be respresented by the following set of frames: ACUTE-GLOMERULONEPHRITIS, GLOMERULITIS, SODIUM-RETENTION, ACUTE-RENAL-FAILURE, ACUTE-HYPERTENSION, RECENT-STREPTOCOCCAL-

INFECTION. Therefore, some means of combining numerical scores must be used, since the "real" score for this hypothesis is divided among these several frames. We have termed the process by which such scores are combined "score-propagation." We approach the problem by organizing the set of frames into a heirarchy, in this case with ACUTE-GLOMERULONEPHRITIS at the apex. Scores are passed along the heirarchy by well-defined rules.

Question Selection

The processes of hypothesis generation and evaluation are both passive, i.e., they do not require additional data from the user. At this point, the active (present illness) and passive (CPC) modes of the program diverge. In the passive mode, an additional finding is provided and the cycle repeats. In the active mode, question selection now occurs. Our current rather naive mechanism for question selection ranks all the active frames by their numerical scores and pursues the frame that has the highest score but which has not yet been established as present in the patient. Pursuit of hypotheses consists of examining the frames associated with those hypotheses and all closely related frames and asking for information which is expected by thoses frames (i.e., the prototypical findings) but which has not yet been specified by the user as being either present or absent. The process continues until all frames are either confirmed (i.e., established as present) or rejected.

PROBLEMS WITH THE PRESENT ILLNESS PROGRAM

The major problems with this program center around its mechanisms for hypothesis evaluation. We shall not make these yet unsolved problems a major part of this discussion since we have chosen to focus on the issue of context formation. However, we might mention the requirements for hypothesis evaluation which will have to be met for that process to form an effective part of any diagnostic system. In most circumstances, neither the physician nor any diagnostic program can establish a diagnosis with certainty. Therefore, it will be necessary to provide measures of belief that can be used as the basis for decisions about diagnostic tests, the termination of the diagnostic phase, and therapeutic decision making. Our group has been interested in decision analysis as a tool for such decision making on the wards, and we therefore find it quite natural to apply these techniques to diagnostic and therapeutic programs.

The use of such techniques requires a measure of belief which is in fact a true probability so that expected values can be calculated. The advantages of such a measure are obvious: much is already known about probability theory, the expected value of information might be calculated and compared to the cost of obtaining that information, thresholds could be established for both ordering tests and terminating the diagnostic phase, and the output of the diagnostic program could be used directly by downstream therapeutic programs. One is therefore tempted to use Bayesian inference in the diagnostic phase; indeed, much of the early work in automated diagnosis focused on those techniques. Unfortunately a problem arises -- those techniques are not applicable in unbounded domains. Many prior discussions of the shortcomings of Bayesian inference have concentrated on the lack of independence of many of the conditional probabilities. This limitation might be solved by massive efforts at data collection, although such efforts often result in a combinatorial explosion of data. Our concern, however, lies at a more basic level. The assumptions which underlie Bayes' rule are completeness and mutual exclusivity in the domain of inference. Although the requirement for completeness can be approached in most practical diagnostic problems, mutual exclusivity is only rarely to be found in the setting of the context formation task which occurs when the physician is presented with the patient's chief complaint. We therefore believe that one should use the techniques of Bayesian inference and decision analysis only after a rather narrow context has been established. Typically, this requires that the problem be narrowed to three or four alternative diagnoses. Of course, several such contexts may exist in parallel, but Bayesian inference can only be applied within a particular context, not between contexts. We are currently investigating a variety of approaches to this context narrowing task -- techniques which do not require the inappropriate use of Bayesian or pseudo-Bayesian inference. These approaches include the limited use of flow charts and discrimination nets and the extension of the concept of triggering. That extension considers the short-term memory to be a smaller long-term memory, from which frames are activated into narrower sub-contexts, i.e., smaller short-term memories. Clearly, these ideas are in a most preliminary form at this time and will require extensive refinement before they become practical. Since this meeting is a "working conference," we do not feel that it is inappropriate to present these ideas so that others might comment on them and help us to refine them.

Yet another problem with the current system concerns its mechanism of context formation. Since the control structure simulates a distributed one and various disease states have been divided into separate, almost atomic frames, we are often faced with an over-abundance of active frames and must therefore take steps to control the proliferation of hypotheses. This problem is further compounded by the aggressive style of hypothesis generation which we have chosen to model. We have made this choice because we feel that such aggressive context formation lies at the root of expertise. The separation of the frames under consideration into active and semi-active states is one mechanism we have used to limit hypothesis proliferation. Recall that the nearby semi-active frame is analogous to having a thought in the back of one's mind. The heuristic programs which we described above are another approach to the limitation of hypothesis generation since they pre-process each finding before it is exposed to the full fury of the short-term memory. Finally, we have used the principle of parsimony to restructure the working context whenever possible by combining separate frames into more coherent hypotheses.

Finally, our approach to question selection is, at best, naive. Certainly heuristic approaches gathered from experts and compiled into data acquisition modules will improve the situation. The ultimate solution to that problem, however, will lie in establishing appropriate measures of belief which will allow the techniques of decision analysis to be used to guide the question selection task.

OTHER APPROACHES TO CONTEXT FORMATION

Having described in perhaps too much detail the approach and limitations of our present illness system, we now turn to other artificial intelligence programs that deal with medical diagnosis and shall comment on some of their approaches to context formation. We shall not consider the flow-charted approaches used for acid-base consultation programs and the like, since context formation there either is not an issue or is not dealt with in any meaningful way. We shall confine our comments to the MYCIN[6] program under development at Stanford (and discussed at this conference), to the CASNET[1] program under development at Rutgers, and to the INTERNIST[5] program under development at the University of Pittsburg.

Both MYCIN and CASNET deal with problem domains that are already fairly narrow (the use of antibiotics and the treatment of glaucoma) and, as such, have little difficulty with context formation. The MYCIN system is a rule-based system which tracks along antecedent-consequent links to establish the diagnosis and recommend appropriate therapy. Its context is established by the mention of an assumed organism, and that context is further narrowed by the evolving characteristics of that organism. The CASNET system consists of multiple planes of causally linked nodes which pass weights of belief along the network. The context is established by a set of nodes corresponding to the various disease states which can affect the eye. Each of these contexts is examined, and appropriate weights are attached. The primary node with the highest weight is pursued.

The INTERNIST system is most like our own in that it deals with the relatively unbounded problem domain of diagnosis in internal medicine. It organizes the various possible diseases into a heirarchy generated as information about each disease is entered. Each disease corresponds to a node in the tree and is described by a set of atomic findings, each having two associated weights: an evoking strength and a measure of frequency. The evoking strength is a semi-quantitative analog of the concept of triggering, while the frequency corresponds to our measure of the fit of the case to the frame. INTERNIST uses a third measure which specifies the severity of each abnormal finding. This measure is subtracted from the score of each disease which does not account for that abnormal finding and therefore is analagous to our measure of the ability of the frame to account for the findings of the case. Finally, INTERNIST divides all potential questions into four levels of costliness (e.g., a liver biopsy is more costly than taking a blood pressure). The program attempts to exhaust as many low cost questions as possible before turning to costly ones.

We shall not attempt to explain the full complexity of the INTERNIST system which now encompasses most of the common diseases in internal medicine and which performs quite well. Rather, we shall focus on INTERNIST's approach to context formation. It uses a partitioning algorithm to establish contexts for comaprisons. That algorithm first assigns a score to each disease under consideration, where that score is a function of the sum of all the evoking strengths assigned to findings known to be present minus the sum of all the frequencies assigned to findings known to be absent minus the sum of the severities of all abnormal findings not explained by the disease. The disease with the highest score is then compared to all other diseases in turn. If the combination of these two diseases can explain more of the serious abnormal findings than can either alone, then the two diagnoses are complementary. If the combination does not do better than either alone, then the two diagnoses are alternatives. The set of all alternative diagnoses forms the context for further exploration. Since these alternatives are most often functionally exclusive, it is reasonable to apply Bayesian inference within these contexts. INTERNIST is indeed a performance system and can be quite impressive. Its major problem lies with its inability to deal effectively with cases that cut across organ system boundaries (e.g., the collagen diseases) so that mutual exclusivity does not hold.

CONCLUSIONS

We have described a computer system which embodies some theories of clinical cognition. This system has allowed us to examine the issue of context formation and has resulted in the idea that triggering can be used to establish contexts for subsequent clinical reasoning. We have discussed some limitations in this system which relate to our inadequate understanding of hypothesis evaluation and have pointed toward several promising approaches to this problem. We hope that continued work in this area will eventually help to achieve three goals: first, the development of a computer system that can provide expert consultations to clinicians in remote areas where such consultations are not now available; second, the development of a better understanding of expert clinical reasoning that will allow us to better teach our medical students and young physicians; third, the development of an understanding of problem-solving techniques that will further the field of artificial intelligence and thereby find application in other field of human endeavor, far removed from clinical medicine.

REFERENCES

1. Kulikowski CA, Weiss S, Safir A:
   Glaucoma diagnosis and therapy by computer.
   Proc Ann Mtg Assoc Res in Vision and Ophthalmol, Sarasota, Florida, 1973.

2. Minsky M:
   A framework for representing knowledge.
   The Psychology of Computer Vision (Winston PH, ed),
     New York, McGraw-Hill, 1975.

3. Moon D:
   MACLISP Reference Manual.
   Project MAC, Massachusetts Institute of Technology, Cambridge, 1974.

4. Pauker SG, Gorry GA, Kassirer JP, Schwartz WB:
   Towards the simulation of clinical cognition.
   Amer Journ Med 60:981-996, 1976.

5. Pople H, Werner G:
   An information processing approach to theory formation in biomedical research
   Proc AFIPS Spring Joint Computer Conf, p1125, 1972.

6. Shortliffe EH:
   Computer-based medical consultations: MYCIN.
   New York, Elsevier, 1976.

7. Sussman GJ, McDermott DV:
   From PLANNER to CONNIVER -- a genetic approach.
   Proc AFIPS Fall Joint Computer Conf, Anaheim Calif, p1171, 1972.

8. Szolovits P, Hawkinson LB, Martin WA:
   An overview of OWL, a language for knowledge representation.
   (submitted for publication).

Computational Linguistics in Medicine, Schneider/Sagvall Hein, eds.
North-Holland Publishing Company, (1977)

SYSTEMATIZATION IN THE REGISTRATION
OF MEDICAL DIAGNOSTIC STATEMENTS

J. van Egmond, L. Decoussemaker and R. Wieme
Department of Medical Informatics
University Hospital of Gent
Gent, Belgium

In order to register in a medical record the complex medical reality expressed by the physician's statements concerning a patient's health condition, it is proposed to define the "diagnostic conclusion" as being a set of working
diagnoses concerning each problem of a patient. These
working diagnoses - formulated whenever a statement is
needed as a basis for a decision for a care action - are
interrelated by "secondary to", are modulated by the indication "secondary to a diagnosis" or "secondary to a procedure for a diagnosis". The last working diagnoses in a
diagnostic conclusion express the final diagnoses a physician
considers for the patient's problem.

An analysis of the application of this linguistic model in the
computerized medical record system COMPADOS of the
University Hospital of Gent demonstrates that its use is
feasible in routine practice and that it fulfils, in a satisfactory way, the needs of the clinicians for registration
and processing of their diagnostic statements.

INTRODUCTION

As the formulation by a physician of a diagnosis (1, 2) not only depends on
his medical practice, on his knowledge of the patient's health condition and
of the nature of the disease underlying the label he is expressing, but also
on his educational maturity and cultural level, the elaboration of a linguistic
model which reflects the physician's natural language is very complex.

In fact the model should be able to formalize in a structured way the complex medical reality a physician is considering by his diagnostic statements
(3).

A study of the medical practice in a university hospital resulted in several
basic concepts for a linguistic model, which now is applied to the regular
registration of diagnoses in the hospital. The detailed description and analysis of the results of the implementation show that the system is feasible
in the patient care oriented medical record system (COMPADOS) of the hospital (4).

A LINGUISTIC MODEL FOR A SYSTEMATIZATION IN THE REGISTRATION OF MEDICAL DIAGNOSTIC STATEMENTS

Analysis of medical practice

An analysis of medical practice, performed with the medical records of a
university hospital, shows that the physician, before being able to formulate

a final diagnosis, very often treats a patient on the basis of preliminary diagnoses, the so-called "working diagnoses".

These working diagnoses usually are formulated whenever a concise description of the patient's health status is required for a decision concerning the next therapeutic or diagnostic step. The working diagnoses are oriented towards care-action.

At the moment a physician decides to define the final diagnosis labeling the underlying disease, all working diagnoses can be brought together in a set of working diagnoses interrelated by "secondary to", i.e. the diagnostic conclusion.

This diagnostic conclusion summarizes the physicians consideration concerning a particular problem of the individual patient.

In a medical record all these statements are noted with the respective dates in order to reflect the evolution in time of the patient's health status.

The proposed linguistic model

A "diagnostic conclusion" is defined as being a set of "working diagnoses" - care action oriented diagnostic statements - all related to one "initial working diagnosis" (the diagnostic statement concerning the reason why the patient appeals to the physician). All working diagnoses are interrelated by "secondary to", differentiating whether the diagnosis is secondary to another working diagnosis or is secondary to a diagnostic-therapeutic procedure performed on the basis of a working diagnosis. The underlying disease(s) is (are) expressed by the "final working diagnosis(es)". All working diagnoses formulated between the initial and the final diagnoses are called "intermediate working diagnoses" (Fig. 1).

Figure 1
The diagnostic conclusion : the model and an example

initial working diagnosis   FEVER

← secondary to (specification)   ← secondary to the diagnosis
    intermediate working diagnosis   PNEUMONIA

    ← secondary to (specification)   ← secondary to surgery for
        final diagnosis   ULCER OF STOMACH

← secondary to (specification)   ← secondary to the diagnosis
    intermediate working diagnosis   URINARY TRACT INFECTION

    ← secondary to (specification)   Fig. 1b : Application of the linguis-
        intermediate working diagnosis   tic model for a patient suffering
                                            fever due to a pneumonia, compli-
        ← . . . .   cating surgery for a gastric ulcer,
                                            and due to a urinary tract infection.
← . . . .

Fig. 1a : The linguistic model

A working diagnosis is registered in a two dimensional coding system with "disturbance" and "localization" as parameters. If the causal agent is a microbiological or a chemical factor, a concatenation of the two working diagnoses ('formulation of the patient's condition 'secondary to' the impact of the agent') may result in a three dimensional structure : (disturbance ∏ localization) ◀─ agent (5, 6).

In order to integrate the diagnostic statements into the patient oriented medical record COMPADOS, several other items are also recorded, e.g. date of the start and end of the condition, certainty of the diagnosis, importance of the statement in the medical record,... In order to get around the difficulty of the different semantic contents of a term depending on the feelings of a physician, the identity of the physician and of his medical department is also stored for each working diagnosis.

The validity of the data in the medical record is ensured by input checks at the moment of the introduction into the computer system and by output checks by presenting the registered data on a document to the physician that he inserts after controlling into the medical record of the patient.

ANALYSIS OF THE USE OF THE REGISTRATION SYSTEM

Analysis of the registration process

a. The registering physicians

The participating physicians accept very well the splitting up of a diagnostic statement into its working diagnoses with specification of their relationship. This procedure enables the physician to register diagnostic statements in parallel with the progress of the patient care. The detailed registration of these working diagnoses is useful for patient care itself in case of re-consideration of the patient and permits a very selective retrieval of patients for a scientific study. This model can also be applied as a short-hand written summary of the patient's medical history (Fig. 2).

Figure 2

Application of the model for written medical records

```
            D                    O
fever   ◀────   pneumonia   ◀────   gastric ulcer
            D
        ◀────   urinary tract infection


or
                          D                    D
        1 fever       ◀────  2  and       ◀────  4
                          O
        2 pneumonia   ◀────  3

        3 gastric ulcer

        4 urinary tract infection
```

b. The computerization procedure

The described model enables the Department for Medical Informatics to code all diagnostic statements of the physicians and to store the diagnostic con-

clusions in the medical record system COMPADOS. It must however be recognized that the encoders sometimes have to reformulate the physicians'
statements in order to fit the data into the proposed model.

Analysis of the registered diagnostic conclusions

a. Method

As a diagnostic conclusion may contain a variable number of working diagnoses, a classifying system for the diagnostic conclusions had to be elaborated
in order to facilitate the analysis of the registered diagnostic conclusions.

A diagnostic conclusion can be considered to have a hierarchic tree-structure,
starting from the initial working diagnosis, branching to the intermediate working diagnoses and reaching at the end the final diagnoses. The operators
"secondary to" delimit levels of the same distance from the initial working
diagnosis. In this way each diagnostic conclusion may be labeled by the
number of levels of working diagnoses it contains.

In order to differentiate the diagnostic conclusions of the same number of
levels, the maximum number of working diagnoses which refer on this level
to the same working diagnosis on a previous level will also be indicated
(Fig. 3).

Figure 3
Schematic representation of the application of the classification system for diagnostic conclusions. Examples.

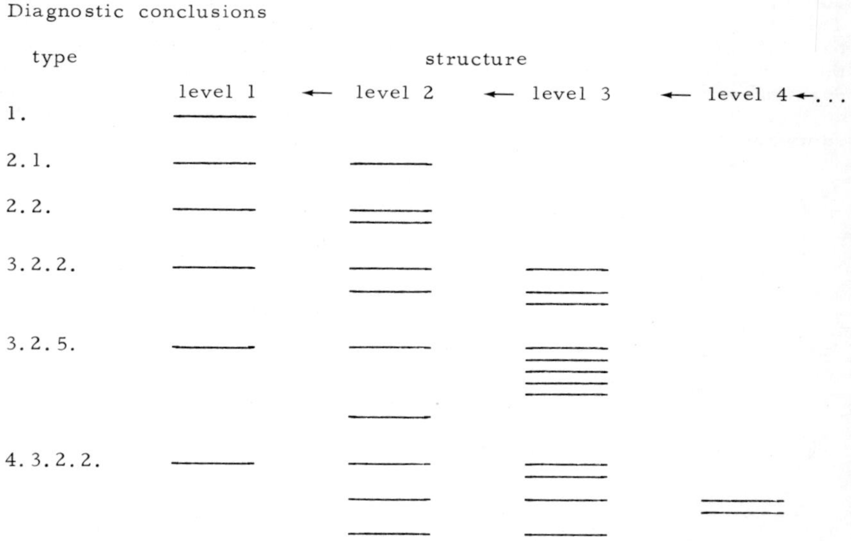

Diagnostic conclusions

The classifying label expresses not only the number of levels in the diagnostic conclusion but also the maximum number of working diagnoses possible
on each level of the diagnostic conclusion.

In a final step a diagnostic conclusion is defined by the contents of each working diagnosis and by the relation between the working diagnoses (secondary to a diagnosis, secondary to a procedure for a diagnosis).

b. Results

An analysis of the diagnostic conclusions, registered for 6.490 patients treated in the internal and surgical departments of the university hospital, is shown in table 1 and Fig. 4.

Table 1

Analysis of the diagnostic conclusions of 6490 patients

Diagnostic conclusions	Frequency				
Type	All (1)		Different (2)		Elimination (3)
	n	%	n	%	%
Type 1	15737	74.23	3889	47.41	75.29
1.0.0.0.0.	15737	74.23	3889	47.41	75.29
Type 2	4664	22.00	3519	42.90	24.55
2.1.0.0.0.	4488	21.17	3345	40.78	25.47
2.2.0.0.0.	146	0.69	144	1.76	1.37
2.3.0.0.0.	16	0.08	16	0.20	0.00
2.4.0.0.0.	14	0.07	14	0.17	0.00
Type 3	653	3.08	650	7.92	0.46
3.1.1.0.0.	558	2.63	555	6.77	0.54
3.1.2.0.0.	13	0.06	13	0.16	0.00
3.1.3.0.0.	2	0.01	2	0.02	0.00
3.1.4.0.0.	1	0.01	1	0.01	0.00
3.2.1.0.0.	67	0.32	67	0.82	0.00
3.2.4.0.0.	2	0.01	2	0.02	0.00
3.3.1.0.0.	8	0.04	8	0.10	0.00
3.3.2.0.0.	1	0.01	1	0.01	0.00
3.4.1.0.0.	1	0.01	1	0.01	0.00

Table continued

Diagnostic conclusions	Frequency				
Type	All (1)		Different (2)		Elimination (3)
	n	%	n	%	%
Type 4	130	0. 61	130	1. 58	0. 00
4.1.1.1.0.	106	0. 50	106	1. 29	0. 00
4.1.1.2.0.	2	0. 01	2	0. 02	0. 00
4.1.1.3.0.	1	0. 01	1	0. 01	0. 00
4.1.2.1.0.	8	0. 04	8	0. 10	0. 00
4.1.3.1.0.	1	0. 01	1	0. 01	0. 00
4.1.4.1.0.	2	0. 01	2	0. 02	0. 00
4.2.1.1.0.	6	0. 03	6	0. 07	0. 00
4.2.2.1.0.	1	0. 01	1	0. 01	0. 00
4.3.1.1.0.	3	0. 01	3	0. 04	0. 00
Type 5	15	0. 07	15	0. 18	0. 00
5.1.1.1.1.	12	0. 06	12	0. 15	0. 00
5.1.1.1.2.	2	0. 01	2	0. 02	0. 00
5.2.1.1.1.	1	0. 01	1	0. 01	0. 00
Total	21199	100. 00	8203	100. 00	61. 30

(1) Frequency of all diagnostic conclusions without the elimination of identical Diagnostic conclusions.
(2) Frequency of the different diagnostic conclusions after elimination of identical Diagnostic conclusions.
(3) Reduction of the number of diagnostic conclusions due to the elimination of the identical Diagnostic conclusions.

Figure 4
The diagnostic conclusions for 6490 patients

number of patients   : 6490
number of diagnostic conclusions : 21199
number of working diagnoses   : 28229

→   diagnostic conclusions/patient   : 3. 27
      working diagnoses/patient   : 4. 35
      working diagnoses/diagnostic conclusion   : 1. 33

Table 2 and Fig. 5 demonstrate the results of the same type of analysis, performed on the diagnostic conclusions of two well-characterized departments : a department of intensive care and a department of endocrinology.

c. Discussion

→ Most of the registered diagnostic conclusions belong to the one-level type (type 1) (74 %). Even for the multilevel types the physicians feel that the

interrelation between working diagnoses is an acceptable method for the registration of their considerations. It may be stressed that diagnostic conclusions with several final diagnoses (underlying diseases) are quite common
(1.46 %).

→ It is striking that the higher level diagnostic conclusions are much more
differentiated (small reduction (21 %) of the number of diagnostic conclusions when eliminating identical diagnostic conclusions) than the type 1 diagnostic conclusions (considerable reduction (75 %) of the number of diagnostic conclusions when eliminating the identical ones). Considering only the
different diagnostic conclusions, a large percentage (52 %) of these diagnostic conclusions is composed of the higher level diagnostic conclusions.

These facts may indicate that the higher the level of the diagnostic conclusion, the more it is patient specific.

→ A density study, i.e. a study of the number of observed working diagnoses in relation to the possible number of working diagnoses in a given type
of diagnostic conclusion, indicates that the higher level diagnostic conclusions
not always contain all working diagnoses that could fit into the structure
(type 1 : 100 %, type 2 : 100 %, type 3 : 97.2 %, type 4 : 96.8 %, type 5:
96.3 %).

→ From an analysis (see table 2 and Fig. 5) the differences in the frequency of the types of the diagnostic conclusions encountered in the intensive care
department and in the endocrinology ward, it appears that in both wards the
registration is quite similar although the patients in the intensive care department only stay for the intensive treatment and not for the long investiga-
tive and care period as they do in a ward of internal medicine.

Figure 5

The comparison of the registration in two medical departments

	intensive care	endocrinology
number of patients	1045	2225
number of diagnostic conclusions	2116	6094
number of working diagnoses	2670	7902
diagnostic conclusions/patient	2.02	2.74
working diagnoses/patient	2.56	3.55
working diagnoses/diagnostic conclusion	1.26	1.30

Table 2
Comparison of the registration in two different medical departments

Diagnostic conclusions Type	Intensive Care		Endocrinology	
	Frequency			
	All %	Different %	All %	Different %
Type 1	79.87	53.55	74.18	53.43
Type 2	16.97	37.94	22.12	37.32
2.1.0.0.0.	16.02	35.41	21.00	34.65
2.2.0.0.0.	0.76	2.03	0.87	2.07
2.3.0.0.0.	0.19	0.51	0.10	0.24
2.4.0.0.0.	0.00	0.00	0.15	0.37
Type 3	2.46	6.60	3.36	8.32
3.1.1.0.0.	2.17	5.84	2.89	7.14
3.1.2.0.0.	0.05	0.13	0.02	0.04
3.1.3.0.0.	0.00	0.00	0.02	0.04
3.1.4.0.0.	0.00	0.00	0.02	0.04
3.2.1.0.0.	0.24	0.63	0.33	0.81
3.2.4.0.0.	0.00	0.00	0.03	0.08
3.3.1.0.0.	0.00	0.00	0.07	0.16
Type 4	0.47	1.27	0.34	0.85
4.1.1.1.0.	0.33	0.89	0.28	0.69
4.1.1.2.0.	0.00	0.00	0.02	0.04
4.1.1.3.0.	0.00	0.00	0.02	0.04
4.1.3.1.0.	0.00	0.00	0.02	0.04
4.2.1.1.0.	0.05	0.13	0.02	0.04
4.3.1.1.0.	0.09	0.25	0.00	0.00
Type 5	0.24	0.63	0.03	0.08
5.1.1.1.1.	0.14	0.38	0.03	0.08
5.1.1.1.2.	0.05	0.13	0.00	0.00
5.2.1.1.1.	0.05	0.13	0.00	0.00
Total	n = 2116	n = 788	n = 6094	n = 2465

Use of the system for statistical purposes

As the primary goal of the registration system is to be useful for patient care, - as is the formulation of physicians concerning a patient - it tends to contain mainly very specific information : each individual patient possibly can have his own diagnoses. In this way the registered information does not lend itself very well to the elaboration of statistical surveys. In order to realize these statistics a translation system has to be involved, which translates the specific and detailed diagnostic conclusions into general statistical data.

CONCLUSION

The definition of a diagnostic conclusion as a set of interrelated working diagnoses seems to be a workable approach to the systematization of the registration of the complex medical reality as expressed by the clinicians' natural language statements.

The analysis of the proposed model demonstrates that the clinicians of a university hospital can easily formulate the diagnostic statements in the frame of the model and that the registered data satisfy the medical needs in the hospital.

References

(1) R.L. Engle and B.J. Davis : Medical diagnosis : present, past and future, Arch. Int. Med. 112 (1963) 512-543.
(2) A.R. Feinstein : Clinical Judgment, (The Wilkins and Wilkins Co. 1967).
(3) A.W. Pratt, M.G. Pacak, M. Epstein and G. Dunham : Computers and natural languages, J. of Clin. Computing III (1973) 85-100.
(4) J. van Egmond, L. Decoussemaker, R.J. Wieme and W. Bossaert : Implementation of an information system for patient care in the University Hospital of Gent, Information Systems for Patient Care, ed. by J. van Egmond, P.F. de Vries Robbé and A.H. Levy (North Holland Publishing Company, Amsterdam, 1976).
(5) J. van Egmond and R.J. Wieme : Systematized codification of medical diagnostic statements, Medinfo 74, ed. by J. Anderson and M. Forsythe (North Holland Publishing Company, Amsterdam, 1974) 931-933.
(6) J. van Egmond and R.J. Wieme : Coding diagnosis of medical records : a challenge, J. of Clin. Computing III (1973) 130-135.

Computational Linguistics in Medicine, Schneider/Sagvall Hein, eds.
North-Holland Publishing Company, (1977)

REMEDE : AN ARTIFICIAL LANGUAGE
FOR CLINICAL DOCUMENTATION

M. de HEAULME, Ch. MERY
INSERM U 88
91, bd de l'hôpital
75634 PARIS CEDEX 13

REMEDE is an example of a class of "context-calculable" documentation languages using an organized thesaurus of current medical
words and a set of logical operators which are not necessarily
boolean.

Due to its logical construction, no formal silence occurs during
interrogation (the only one comes from implicit content of users'
requests), and noise is considerably reduced.

Tested since 1974 in Rheumatology, and completely studied for
applications in Endocrinology, Urology and Vascular Surgery, the
way opened by REMEDE seems efficient for most clinical documentary
activities aiming at report processing, bibliography and documentary aid on academical descriptions of illnesses.

I -   Other papers (1, 2, 3, 4) have detailled the reasons which have led to define REMEDE, an artificial language for medical documentation.

Briefly they are :

- in medicine, notions having to be described are so variable and their number so
  large that even inside one speciality, descriptive techniques working by enumera-
  tion of pre-defined items lead to improper tools when the field is not limited
  and clearly defined ;
- usual combinatory techniques are convenient, but key words techniques successfully employed when they are applied to bibliography,are no longer sufficient for
  clinical descriptions, for they provide too much noise or silence ;
- natural language is not ready to be usually processed yet ;
- medical requests may be very complex, however, the power of interrogating depends
  on the richness of links described between data, including temporal links ;
- using a documentation system on computer has a sense only if physicians can interrogate data as often as they want, however physicians proceed step-by-step in
  their documentary research. Consequently, the system must be very effective and
  the cost of each question very low.
- But in any case, using combinatory descriptive techniques presents a danger : as
  each physician indexes the information from his own point of view, a common reference is missing, and data are not completely normalized. Consequently results
  coming from documentation systems could not be relevant for scientific working,
  if standard procedures of collecting data are not overimposed to each description.

In fact, the clinical activity seems to require a two-levels system : a general documentation level working as a reservoir of information and dealing with combinatory techniques of description, and a specific level where items must have been strictly pre-defined, either for patient administration or for scientific working.

The proportion of each level depends on each application type and moves on time.
REMEDE, as a system, provides a heading containing normalized items corresponding to
each application, followed by reports written with an artificial language.

Three aims dealing with clinical documentation are pursued, in attempt to provide
facilities :

- for writing any kind of medical reports, as typically are discharge summaries ;
- for making specialized medical bibliography (instead of general systems as MEDLARS, Erxcepta Medica, etc ...). Here the heading items contain paper references, and the text describes the paper content. The system is convenient for services or medical associations which have their own lecturers and their own specialized abstracts.
- for asking a medical data base of illnesses. The academical tableaus are reported instead of patients or papers, and the system becomes an aide-mémoire for physicians.

In all cases, the main problem is to retrieve very specific and sensitive results, as far as silence cannot be tolerated in Medicine, and noise must remain very little in the daily medical usage, contrary to what is accepted in current bibliography.

II - LINGUISTIC ASPECTS

As the interrogation power depends on the data structure, causes of noise and silence must be analyzed both in relation to semantic and syntaxic properties of the language.

1. Semantic structure

It has been recognized today, that a unique lexical organization of the words could not remain convenient for all the words of a general thesaurus. Each semantic dimension of the field has its original structure. For example, if symptoms are classified from a certain point of view, this classification is no longer relevant for simultaneously classifying either etiologies or topographies and so forth.

This fact is at the origin of a lot of problems met in nomenclature usage since each word compounding one item label belongs to its own semantic structure, meanwhile the whole item is classified itself according to the nomenclature aim. But if elementary words (included compounded-words) are now independently classified according to each semantic dimension, a very important property appears : they can be ordered each other according to one simple hierarchy naturally defined, and easily accepted by all users.

Moreover, the rank of a word in its hierarchy defines exactly its precision for users and the computer processing as well.

If such a solution is not taken, description of semantic linkages between words becomes inextricable because each word belongs to different organizations, which all have to be taken into account simultaneously. One can see immediatly how an important part of the "sensible" side of a language is related to the fact that words have to be interpreted differently depending on their semantic situation.

On the contrary, when the adopted solution is separated classes of terms, the meaning of a word is immediatly defined by its rank in its own hierarchy, related to the other words of the same class, however relations to the other word classes will be achieved by syntax relations and no longer by lexical definitions.

Solutions are acceptable if the classes definition is natural to users. In the actual REMEDE, 7 classes have been retained : symptoms (or signs), topographies, etiologies,treatments, examinations, results (of a treatment or an examination) and adjectives. This choice will be discussed later,but if required,other classes could be added without making the system unacceptable. As usual, an only formal solution cannot avoid misunderstanding or misusage of words. It appears quickly that these difficulties concern above all the etiology   class - symptoms as "white tongue" are perfectly recognized for centuries, and topographies as well. But etiologies may be understood in different ways by different physicians, renewing the language sensibility. "Chronic bronchitis" has not the same meaning for specialists and

general practitioners , "illness of X..." does not always imply the same medical
content for all physicians, etc ... Nosography contains a lot of terms or expressions having a precise sense only for one school or one group of physicians.

Finally, words of this class may have different meanings, or the same meaning may
be expressed by different words. Most current difficulties in indexing or retrieving come from this nosological variability and leads to an unacceptable sensibility of the language. Solution is to have put these words out of the thesaurus into
a users' manual showing how they must explicitely be written with REMEDE.

Thus,only elementary words well understood by all users are retained, and reports
are made by describing all the exact elementary signs related to precise causes.
Also this way appears as the only one which enables the computer to decide perti-
nently if words are relevant to a question. On the contrary case, the computer
would have to know the implicit information contained in the label "illness of X..".
Moreover, many patients never have the complete set of signs academically described
and/or may present other signs.

Finally, the previous choices represent the semantic constraints which allow to limit the semantic variability and thus to define clearly what it could be expected
from interrogations. For the moment these constraints are well-accepted by all
users, and will not be moved until other procedures permit to squeeze the semantic
sensibility.

2. Syntaxic structure

Syntaxic causes of noise and silence consist in lack of specific linkages between
words. For example, using keywords   with only simple juxtaposition of
words "cancer kidney, superior pole, ablation" cannot lead to decide if the cancer
or the ablation concerns the whole kidney or its superior pole only. This difficulty is clearly different from confusing   semantic relations.

2.1. Grammatical operators

The problem is now to define the nature of the needed prepositions. Only two properties are required in order to construct a documentation language processed by
computers :

a. The constructed grammar has to be factorisable. It is not only a formal requirement but allows the user to build complex sentences, or, if he cannot (or would
   not, or is not capable of ...), to make the same description by juxtaposition of
   simple sentences easier to write. Taking the arithmetic syntax for example,
   A ✳ (B (C+D)) is strictly equivalent to ABC + ABD
   The only difference is that the simplest way needs a certain redundancy of terms.
   Here A and B have to be written twice in the second form.
b. Sentences must have only one meaning, that is to say relations noted by the language prepositions must be univocal logical operators. This can be reached by
   algorithms and not only by boolean calculation. This point merits to be discussed, in relation to the importance of its consequences.

Most artificial languages basically use the facilities offered by the computer technology to process directly boolean operators. But this fact is also related to the
"context-free" constitution of these languages. No other relations have to disturb
the calculation, which means also that no semantic variability of variables is able
to be taken into account,except if it can be expressed itself by a boolean calculation.

When variables to be processed are formally defined by users, or univocally identify the represented objects, no problem occurs as it is the case in management,
scientific calculation, process control, etc ...

But when the variables are the words of a natural language, they have a great semantic sensibility. Then documentation languages using only boolean syntax

necessarily lead to noise and silence coming from the underlying semantic relations which are ignored by the processing, if they are not by the user. The difficulty is at its top when documents belong to different natural languages which have each their own structure, as it is the case in general bibliography.

But bibliography has first to identify document. Moreover, users interrogate few times each year. Danger to miss documents can be overcome by other techniques, as crossed references, and, anyway, is not immediatly damaging for people health.

In clinical documentation the interest is the content analysis of the document, some serious consequences may appear, coming from insufficient or wrong results, and interrogations must be as frequent as the staff needs, which implies a very effective processing for avoiding hours of verification.

It has been said above how the semantic variability is squeezed in REMEDE by the thesaurus organization in separated classes of terms. But the relations existing between these classes have not been taken into account yet, and are going to be achieved syntaxically.

Summarizing these relations, it appears immediatly that some of them cannot be exactly reduced to boolean operators as "attached to", "treated by", "due to" or "related to", etc ... If only boolean operators as implication are taken instead of them, noise and silence appear again and/or the natural meaning of sentences disappears.

But as long as computers also allow to process algorithms, nothing forbids to define proper functions which will be processed as syntaxic non-boolean operators, and to construct the automate of such a language. The system will be successful as far as these operators will conserve a univocal meaning.

The last problem is to know if the number of such operators is small enough in Medicine for providing a sufficiently simple language or, in other words, if current medical sentences have some basic structures.

Until today, the following operators defined in 1972, have resisted time and their application in Rheumatogoly, Endocrinology, Urology, Vascular Surgery too :

Symbols	operators	meaning
$<$	"of"	linking a term to a topography exclusively
$>$	"due to"	designing cause/effect relation
$*$	"treated by"	attaching treatments to description
$=$	"equal"	introducing results of a treatment or of an examination.

If there are S for Symptoms, T for Topographies, E for Etiology, TR for TReatments and R for Results, the basic clinical sentence is : $S < T > E * TR = R$

Introducing now the comma "," for "AND" and the natural usage of brackets the following sentences are allowed : $S_1, S_2, S_3 \ldots \quad < \quad T_1, T_2, T_3 \ldots \quad > \quad E_1$

(a) - $S_1, \ldots < T_1 > E < T_2$

(b) - $S_1, \ldots < T_1, \ldots > E_1 \; > \; E_2 \ldots$

   - $(S_1, S_2) < T_1 > E_1 > E_2 < T_2, T_3 \ldots$

   - $(S_1 < T_1 * TR_1 = ++), (S_2 < T_2 * TR_2 = -), \ldots > E_1$

   - $S_1, S_2, \ldots < (T_1 * TR_1), (T_2 * TR_2), \ldots > E_1$

   - $S_1 < T_1 > E_1 * TR_1$

   - etc ...

One can see (a) that one etiology is reputed to have the topographies located at
his left until other topographies specify it. Etiologies can also be chained (b),
what solves the problem to design complications specifically.

More complex writing is allowed with multiple brackets, but most physicians prefer
to repeat some terms and write simple sentences.

Other operators must be added to this basic set :

/	"juxtaposition"	introducing independent sentences
%	"between"	binds some bipolar topographies (anastomosis, fistulae, etc ...)
—	"qualified by"	links adjectives to names

Some of these adjectives are named "modifiers" because they have a specific use :

. right, left, bilateral are respectively written - R, - L, - B
. Doubtful is noted - ?
. certain is noted - ↑
. No is noted - N (meaning "absent" and allowing to index negative signs).

2.2. Time indexation

Each event is preceeded by a time indication, according to the following rules :

"date"   ponctual event
"date - "   beginning date
" - date"   ending date
"date 1 - date 2"   dates concerning a whole episode

The rule is that each event dated with a beginning date is still running until it
is not closed by a further ending date. If only a part of the dated event is ending,
this part must be repeated and preceeded by the corresponding ending date.

"080773 -" pain, fever > illness X
"- 120773" fever > illness X

This way is necessary as far as computers require completely explicited statements.
"End of illness X" would not have been sufficient for separating different cases
when the illness is ended but not the pain for example, or when several diseases
can deliver the   same symptoms.

One can see that dates play the same role as the juxtaposition operator "/", adding
a temporal meaning to it.

2.3. Other rules

a. P (personal) or F (family) are written inside two double quotes as dates are for
   designing sentences concerning antecedents : "P 0658 -" diabetes mellitus
b. free comments are allowed anywhere between square brackets for precising information or combinations. This facility is very useful for completing a record,
   and save all what escaped the language possibilites.
c. Thesaurus changing is allowed by calling a new thesaurus. The operator is &
   followed by the name of the new speciality and ":"   : ... & CARDIO: ....
   will enter the thesaurus of Cardiology.

Thus a document can be indexed with the most precise words concerning a speciality
without changing anything else in the language or in the execution programs.

Samely, using words of different natural languages presents no   difficulty as
far as the same medical notions have been referred to the same thesaurus code.

The following sentences show how REMEDE is used (heading is not shown) :

    "P75"   pain < knee-L, hip-G

    "0276-0876"   arthritis < knee-L, elbow-G, hip-G > rhumatoid arthritis
                              ✳ gold salts
    "0876"   proteinuria > gold salts
    "1176-"   rhumatoid arthritis ✳ corticoids/ESR=+/
                      Wahler Rose=+/ (Uric acid, white cells)=N
    "0277"   arthritis < hip-G ✳ prothesis

NB : "=N" means the result is "normal"

Finally REMEDE is not "context-free" but remains "context-calculable". This property is obtained both from the thesaurus organization and the syntaxic operator definition. For example the preposition "due to" could mean "related to" or "according
to" as well, as it is the actual case when it is written :
STENOSIS < FEMORAL ART. > ARTERIOGRAPHY
ARTERIOGRAPHY is not a medical etiology, but no confusion occurs at the interrogation step. If difficulties appear, a new class of terms concerned with "circumstances" could be created and would suppress the ambiguity by lexical way. However, if
it was absolutely necessary a new operator as "related to" and noted ":" could
also be created :

STENOSIS < FEMORAL ART. : ARTERIOGRAPHY   or   ARTERIOGRAPHY : STENOSIS < FEMORAL ART.

giving a strictly univocal interpretation to terms. But some circumstances have
also a temporal meaning : hospitalisation, operation, consultation etc ... are multiple, and one must be able to interrogate on the occurence of each one.

Thus the new operator would have to delimit the whole set of sentences related to
a given circumstance, and also to be nested :

"date-date" Hospitalisation I :
               "date"   arteriographyI : stenosis femoral art., etc ...
               "date"   operationI
"date" consultation : .....
"date" consultation : .....
"date-date" hospitalisationII : ...
               "date" arteriographyII : ....
               "date" operationII : ....

One can see how the temporal meaning of circumstances is identified here lexically
(hospitalisationI, HospitalisationII, etc ...). However, they also could have been
indexed by a numerical index 1, 2, 3 ... hospitalisation (1), hospitalisation (2),
etc ... This way would have given a much more sophisticated language, but also a
much more complex one.

This example shows how new functions can be implemented after the semantic and the
syntaxic possibilities of representing them have been discussed.

III. <u>INTERROGATION</u>

Sophistication of language at the indexing step succeeds only if it offers a better
interrogation. With REMEDE, the noise diminishes considerably, the question may be
more precise and relevant, and <u>the logical silence does not exist</u>, as far as the
language is logical and no implicit notions are understated by users.

Different new possibilities have had to be introduced in the query language :

a. the classical AND, OR, NO (equivalent to WITHOUT or EXCEPTED) may be used between terms or brackets
b. dates can also be defined between two boundaries :

"BEG 0175-0176 END 0176-0177" will define events having begun in 1975 and ended during the year 1976.

c. duration can be asked in days (D), months (M) and years (Y). The current time is designed by "."
   "0376-.8M)' designs events having begun in March 1976 and having 8 months ".1Y" designs events having 1 year since the first date they have been meet.

d. questions may be asked ON previous selected files. This way deals with the step-by-step procedure of interrogating usually required by physicians. Moreover, it avoids to make very complex interrogation sentences with multiple brackets and boolean prepositions.

e. selected records can be sorted from heading items values (by sex, age, district, etc ...)

f. one current request in documentation is to search systematically all the existing combinations of a given term class. For example : "list all the treatments concerning ... " (here a sentence defining the clinical situation). The required items are merely replaced in the question sentence by COMB (COMBine)

$$S_1 \ \ldots\ < T_1 \ \ldots\ > E \ \text{\ast\ COMB}$$
samely : $$S_1 \ \ldots\ < T_1 \ \ldots\ > \text{COMB}$$
$$S_1 \ \ldots\ < \text{COMB} > E$$
$$\text{COMB} \ < T_1 \ \ldots\ > E$$

Found terms are printed according to their respective hierarchical rank, with their number of occurences and their percentage. The same could be done ON previously selected files, sorted by age and sex, etc ...

IV. <u>TECHNICAL ASPECTS</u>

It must be discussed if implementation of languages such REMEDE raises new technical problems. Remembering that each interrogation must be rapid and cheap enough for being acceptable during the daily medical activity, the main problem is how to design the record access and how to realize the content analysis of a document as far as possible.

a. Thesaurus organization leads to define a hierarchic code for each term. Solution has been to pre-code record files for interrogation. Thus data are stored in two files : one litteral for simple retrieval, and one coded for interrogating.

   This way offers several interests :

   - direct interrogation on litteral texts would imply to decode each term each time. Pre-coded files have just to be interpreted.
   - only records completely verified are coded. Updating do not interfere with interrogating. Newly updated records are entirely verified and recoded.
   - the size of the coded file is about 1/3 of the litteral one.

     The coded file is sequentially indexed from the record number. Finally with the actual version one interrogation takes about 20 milli-seconds c.p.u. time per record and could be improved.
   - this way is very flexible for introducing new codes, new hierarchy and new prepositions. Recoding the whole litteral source gives the correct new coded file in one pass for ever.

b. But each record has to be entirely processed before knowing if it is relevant to a question. Is it possible to access quicker to relevant records ?

   The classical solutions by inversed files cannot be used directly :

   - they would suppose that selection on <u>index</u>   <u>only</u> would reflect exactly the same selection on records <u>entirely examined</u>. It implies that both index and text would have to be completely context-free themselves, which is not the case here in as much as chronological relations are context sensible too. Thus all the records content itself must be analyzed each time.

In fact inversed files using high-level terms of thesaurus are utilized in order to determine roughly the relevant records which then are analyzed one by one.

One cannot see either how relational techniques could directly overcome the same problem.
c. Such a language must obviously be written in Assembler (now Macro-X from Digital Equipment).   However, text analysis can be performed to day by different high level languages, and solutions as REMEDE could be written for example under MUMPS.
d. The actual version utilizes segmentation and dynamic core allocation. Consequently the execution requires small central core reservation and could be easily implemented on mini-computer.

V. CONCLUSION

REMEDE is an exemple of a class of artificial languages which seems well adapted to clinical documentation, even some adjustments had to be performed for defininga better tool. Complete formalization of such languages has still to be done, but the prototype has shown its feasability, flexibility and acceptability for 3 years in a medical environment. The whole system must include standardized items also, which are always necessary for collecting certain types of medical information.

But more than a system, solutions as REMEDE allow also to possess a unique tool for a large scale of medical activity, including reporting, bibliography and documentary diagnostic aid.

The coming of such languages will permit to make economy on system development and maintenance, and to train more easily the medical staff in computer using. An other point has not been developed in the paper : REMEDE has also a pedagogical virtue, due to the necessity for students or doctors as well to reflect on the precise sense of the words they use, and on how they are exactly inter-related in medical sentences.

One can also see how clinical documentation development is a global strategy for introducing and/or developing computers activities in Medicine at a daily medical level, which seems to be a necessary condition for motivating students and doctors to adapt progressively their mind and their habits to the computer usage.

REFERENCES

(1) de HEAULME, M., MERY, Ch. : REMAID: REsumés Médicaux Archivés et Interrogés Directement par ordinateur. Rev. Inf. Med. 4 (4) 209-218, 1973
(2) de HEAULME, M., MERY, Ch. : REMAID, an artificial language for medical reports on computer. Proceedings of MEDINFO 74, p. 935-941
(3) MERY, Ch., MENKES, C.J., de HEAULME, M., DELBARRE, F. : langage artificiel permettant la mise sur ordinateur d'observations résumées. Rev. du Rhumatisme, 42 (5), 317-326, 1975
(4) de HEAULME, M., MERY, Ch.; Proceedings of MEDCOMP 77, p. 323-338 : Physicians -computer communication.

M. de HEAULME : INSERM U 88, 91, bd de l'Hôpital - F-75634 PARIS CEDEX 13
Ch. MERY : Service de Rhumatologie, Hôpital Cochin,27, rue du faubourg St-Jacques
                          75014 PARIS CEDEX 14

PART III

ASPECTS ON HARDWARE AND SOFTWARE
(FACILITIES AND REQUIREMENTS)

Computational Linguistics in Medicine, Schneider/Sågvall Hein, eds.
North-Holland Publishing Company, (1977)

DESIGNING LISP ORIENTED HARDWARE

Jaak Urmi
Informatics Laboratory
Linkoping University
Linkoping, Sweden

When talking about LISP as a tool in artificial intelligence and computational linguistics everybody seems to agree on the usefulness and validity of this tool. When we try to mention LISP as a tool for applications systems to be used in everyday life, you are immediately met by a variety of arguments against it. A sample of the most common arguments might be:

        It's too large a system!
        It's too slow!
        It's expensive!
        Too complex!
        It never works, and when it does, it produces
                too many errors.
        Whats wrong with FORTRAN/COBOL?

Of course many objections are relevant, and there are some particular problem areas which I would like to address, namely:

SIZE:

The size of systems written in LISP tend to be very large.
This is not a property that must be (or even is) inherent or typical of LISP as such, but rather an effect of the complexity and need for large amounts of information in the problem domains where LISP is traditionally used.

SPEED:

Most systems written in LISP tend to be slow.
This is partly because of the size problem and partly because we have very few LISP systems around that could claim to have a "professional" quality. The main reason though is probably that we have no computers around which are "ideally" suited for LISP the way most computers are suited for COBOL and FORTRAN, and some (one?) are suited for Algol.

SECURITY:

Most (if not all) LISP systems are very unsecure in the sense that many error conditions are not detected (e.g. taking CDR of a number etc.).
This is partly because LISP is a language which uses very late binding, and thus has to rely on run-time checks to a very large extent. These checks cost time. This fact coupled with the general space and speed problem tend to be enough to make LISP implementors leave these checks out, often with the motivation that "it is an experimental system to be used in a research environment, and anyhow

139

we have all these nice debugging tools.."

        I believe that these are the three main reasons why LISP is
"only" a research tool and has not gained wide acceptance as a
language and tool to be used in production work in spite of its
merits. What these problems lead up to is basically that one needs a
half a million dollar computer to run a LISP-based system that keeps
one user happy if the system is of any significant complexity in
terms of the problem it is running.

        The remedy for these problems is obviously to write better
LISP-systems on better hardware.

Today's hardware is in no sense ideal for LISP, a fact that has long
ago been realized, but with today's ever decreasing cost of hardware
components and a general interest in special purpose computers, a
reevaluation of LISP's position as "only" a research tool is long
overdue.

        Currently there are a number of projects going on in the world
aimed at building special purpose LISP-machines. Some of these are
almost completed (i.e. a prototype "works") and promise to be
successful. There is currently also a large interest in
unconventional approaches, using parallel processor philosophies, but
as (non pure) LISP is not an obvious candidate for parallel
processing, these approaches tend to severely limit or redefine LISP
as a language, and should maybe rather be called lambda calculus
machines or some other name.

        I will not present an overview of all projects going on, nor
will I attempt to referee the work done, but I will rather present
some of my own prejudices and pet ideas on what a LISP machine should
look like and what it should include.

        When it comes to the size problem we have a lot to learn from
the Burroughs B1700 architecture. By this I mean that we have to
start encoding and packing data much more than we have done.
Yes, a lot of work has been done on this for LISP, but it has been
confined to machines with basically either 8 or 16 bit "words" and 8
or 16 bit words are just not optimal for LISP.

        We note that LISP has a number of different types of data
objects which all require different size containers. For instance we
have list pointers whose size should be 20 bits if we will allow 1M
list cells, we have pointers to literal atoms whose size should be 17
bits if we allow a maximum of 128K literal atoms, we might have
string pointers of size 15 bits if we are going to allow a total of
32K characters, where we may want to use 9 bits/character to
represent 512 different characters, etc.

        The point is that today we always have to choose a container
(word) size that is larger than what we really need (i.e. a multiple
of 8 or 16) and thus are wasting space in the container as well as in
all data objects that point to it. (e.g. If you have a byte
addressable machine and list cells consist of 8 bytes then all
pointers to list cells will have their 3 low order bits be zero).

Because of the large amounts of information involved in most of our applications it is mandatory to use virtual memory technique of some sort, and thus space reduction is of the utmost importance. If this packing process is not automated somehow we also place a horrendous burden on the implementor who has to be responsible for all the compromises and kludges he introduces trying to achieve decent space usage.

HOW DO WE MAKE PACKING AUTOMATIC?

One could conceive of a memory that is bit addressable and express all references to it through a set of register pairs (call the pair a Base and Length register). Each pair describes part of memory as follows:

Let the i:th register pair be denoted by $[Bi , Li]$.

Let $C(R)$ denote the contents of register R,

then the register pair $[Bi , Li]$ says that the data stored in our memory starting from bit $C(Bi)$ consists of "words" of length $C(Li)$.

A memory reference will consist of a pair $[D , elt]$ where 'D' references a register pair and 'elt' is a "word" number within the memory region described by the register pair. Thus an address issued as $[i,j]$ would yield a bit address (Ba) and length (Ln) as follows:

$$Ba=C(Bi)+j*C(Li)$$
$$La=C(Li)$$

and we could for instance set up:

$B_0 = 0;$ $L_0 = 20;$ for 20 bit list cells (numbered 0,1,2..)

$B_1 = 20*2^{20};$ $L_1 = 9;$ leaving space for 1M list cells of size 20 bits we define this area to contain 9 bit characters

$B_2 = C(B_1)+N*9;$ $L_2 = 1;$ leaving space for the list cells and 'N' 9 bit characters, we now define an area of 1 bit "words" i.e. a bit table

etc.

Using a memory of this design we could allocate the optimal number of bits for each data object. Note that the size and number of data objects might vary from application to application without reprogramming or even reassembling, and they could also vary dynamically (for instance be changed at garbage collection time). Of course there is still a need for encoding of data as discussed in many of the standard references.

This organization toward more "intelligent" memory structuring without placing restrictions on how the implementor is to use it is a feature I judge as most important for future LISP machines (and other machines too).

There are other more esoteric features that one might wish for in the memory of a LISP machine, such as "demons" to monitor "sensitive" data and also maybe to have parts of memory be associative etc.

The architecture of a LISP machine should be a somewhat modified stack architecture, and I see no reason why we should part drastically from the "spaghetti" stack design proposed by Bobrow-Wegbreit (references).

A very time demanding task in LISP is type checking, weather it is programmed explicitly or done implicitly in the system, and we could use some support for this. It should be noted that type checking is done on pointers to data objects (in most implementations anyhow) and not on the data object itself, so when we discuss type checking, we are not talking about a tagged architecture in the traditional sense.

Another point of very great importance is the design of good instruction sets. Such a set can only be designed if one has a very good knowledge of how LISP works on the lcw level and what the really basic primitives are. To enhance security we must include type checking and validity testing in these low level primitives. In practice it should be impossible to use a primitive on a data object it is not intended for, or in a situation where the operation is not valid.

One question that raises a lot of feelings among LISPers is whether our future LISP machines should consist of only an interpreter or a combination of interpreter and compiler (as most current systems). My feelings on this point are somewhat split, but I fear that we will need super efficient compiling systems if the techniques and methodology developed in the LISP community is to get wide acceptance in the "real world" of applications.

I have very briefly mentioned some of my pet ideas when it comes to LISP oriented hardware and I hope it will raise some discussions, questions and thought.

Let me finish with a word of warning: Let us not overestimate the role of micro programming, unsuitable computers do not become suitable because they are (micro) programmable.

REFERENCES

Bobrow, D.G. and Wegbreit, B. ; A Model and Stack Implementation of
        Multiple Environments.
        Comm. ACM 16,10 (Oct 1973)

Deutch, P.L. ; A LISP Machine with very Compact Programs
        Proc. Third International Joint Conf. on
        Artificial Intelligence, 1973

Greenblatt, R. ; The LISP Machine
        Working paper 79, MIT AI-Lab, Cambridge Mass.

Guzman, A. ; A Parallel Configurable Lisp Machine.
        Vol 7, Serie Naranja: Investigaciones No 7
        University of Mexico(UNAM) Mexico

Hartley, A. LISP Machine Project at Bolt Beranek and Newman Inc.
        Private communication

Knight, T. ; CONS
        MIT AI-Lab 1974 Cambridge Mass.

Lamport, L. ; Garbage Collection with Multiple Processes: An
        Exercice in Parallelism.
        Proc. IEEE 1976 Intnl. Conf. on Parallel Processing

Sandewall, E. ; Programming in an Interactive Environment: The LISP
        Expirience
        Report LiTH-MAT-R-76-9 Informatics Lab. Linkoeping Univ.
        Linkoeping, Sweden

Steele, G.L. Jr. ; Multiprocessing Compactifying Garbage Collection.
        Comm. ACM 18 (Sept 1975)

Urmi, J. ;A Shallow Binding Scheme for Fast Environment Changing in a
        "Spaghetti Stack" Lisp System.
        Report LiTH-MAT-R-76-18 Informatics Lab. Linkoeping Univ.
        Linkoeping, Sweden

Wilner, W.T. ; Burroughs B1700 memory utilization
        Fall Joint Computer Conference 1972

Wilner, W.T. ; Design of the Burroughs B1700
        Fall Joint Computer Conference 1972

Winograd, T. ; Project SEC (Reactive Systems)
        working paper Nov 1974, Stanford University AI-lab.

Winograd, T. ; Breaking the Complexity Barrier Again.
        Proc. SIGIR-SIGPLAN interface meeting, Nov 1973

Computational Linguistics in Medicine, Schneider/Sagvall Hein, eds.
North-Holland Publishing Company, (1977)

A Data Structure Model for a Medical
Information System

K. SAUTER (1)

and

K. APPEL (2), G. GRIESSER (3), M. JAINZ (3),
T. RISCH (4), W. SCHNEIDER (2)

(1) Department of Biometrics and Medical Informatics, Medical
School Hannover, FRG, (2) Uppsala University Data Center, Uppsala,
Sweden, (3) Department of Medical Statistics and Documentation,
University Hospital Kiel, FRG, (4) Datalogilaboratoriet, Department
of Computer Science, University of Uppsala, Uppsala, Sweden.

ABSTRACT

The Ministry of Health and Environmental Control of Berlin is
developing a Health Information System (HIS) on the basis of a
multi-satellite network system, comprising a central, regional,
local and functional unit level. The main part of this paper
describes the conceptual structure of the Common Data Base (CDB) of
HIS with special regard to the patient-oriented medical information
originating from the various institutions of the health care
system. This structure comprises the following five levels:

PATIENT, PROBLEM, CASE, EVENT and ACTIVITY.

Each of the levels represents a node in the structure model. A node
is an entity with a set of attributes or "local properties" being
specified for the respective level, and partly referring to
selected data on inferior levels.

The needs for frequent modifications of the logical and physical
structure of the medical data base during the development of HIS
have initiated the implementation of a DATA MANAGER. The concept of
the DATA MANAGER covers facilities for the development of the data
structure model including its documentation and programming support
for application programs accessing the HIS data base.

The outstanding facilities of the INTERLISP system have been found
to be appropriate for writing this DATA MANAGER.

1.0 INTRODUCTION

The Ministry of Health and Environmental Control of Berlin is
developing a Health Information System (HIS) on the basis of a
multi-satellite network system, comprising a central, regional,
local and functional unit level |1, 2, 7, 12|. This structure is
compatible with the model of a HIS as presented by a special study
group of the International Hospital Federation (IHF) |13|.

Experience shows that complex information systems have to be
developed in an interactive way being characterized by the
definition of the strategical goals, the delimitation and
realization of the subsystems, the verification of the target
system on the basis of the experiences made etc. The requirement of
continuous integration of asynchronously developing EDP projects
necessitates an adaptively proceeding project management.

The same procedure has to be chosen for the structuring
of information. Therefore, it is explicitly assumed that the HIS
data base is permanently changing in its logical and physical
structure. Because of its advanced facilities for representation
and manipulation of logical data structures (e.g. lists and trees)
INTERLISP is especially suited for the development of structure
models. The actual INTERLISP 360/370 implementation to be used has
been developed by the Department of Computer Science, Uppsala
University, and the University Data Center of Uppsala on the basis
of the INTERLISP system, as developed by BBN, Boston, Mass., USA.

The INTERLISP programming system is used as well for the
development of the DATA MANAGER because it supports extensive
symbol processing and manipulation (for instance the processing of
source code) and because it is highly interactive.

2.0 THE BASIC MODEL FOR THE REGIONAL SYSTEM

Essential components of the planned health information system for
Berlin comprise the central and the regional levels |1,2,7,12|,
corresponding to the central index and the historical part of the
Common Data Base (CDB) of the HIS model as described by the IHF
study group |13|. In this chapter a structure model of the
historical part of the CDB of HIS is presented with special regard
to the integration and exchange of patient-oriented medical
information originating from the various institutions of the health
care system |11|. This model is considered to be a conceptual image
of certain aspects of interactions between "patient" and "health
care system".

2.1 The structural hierarchy

The design of the structure model is based on the relationships
between the data and the information needs of the users, which can
be expressed by query types. The historical part of the CDB is -
with regard to the macro structure - in principle of the
hierarchical type and comprises the following levels:
level 1. PATIENT
level 2. PROBLEM
level 3. CASE
level 4. EVENT
level 5. ACTIVITY.

In this structure model, each level represents a node with a set of
"local properties LP (ij)" for this level, and selected pointers PL
(ij) referring to data within hierarchically dependent levels with
summarizing and quick-referring functions. Finally a pointer list
establishes the connection to all dependent nodes of the next lower
level. "Local" should be understood in this context as "related
only to this specific node and describing it".

The following contents have been defined:

2.2 Level 1: PATIENT (PA)

The patient is the most comprehensive logical unit or entity within
the CDB. Structure of level 1:

$$PA(<LP(1i)>, <PR(j)>).$$

The list of local properties LP (1i) comprises mainly patient
identification information.

2.3 Level 2: PROBLEM (PR)

The structural levels 2 through 5 are strongly related to the various patient interactions with the health care system and represent a projection of the different time periods during the life span of a patient - as it has been outlined recently in |9| - on to the sequence of system activities (fig. 1). An entry on level 2 comprises all cases of examination and treatment which are connected to one problem. The relationship between a patient's disease and the associated problem may, but must not necessarily, be an one-to-one mapping |14|. Several ailments may occur at the same time, resulting in an overlapping of health care system activities, related to different problems. Therefore the possibility of associating problems is required.

DEFINITION OF INFORMATION INTERVALS IN MEDICAL INFORMATICS

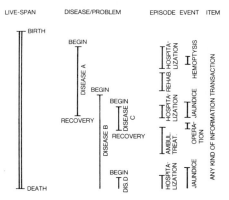

Fig. 1: Definition of patient-oriented information intervals in medical informatics |9|.

Structure of level 2:

PR(<PL(2i)>, <CA(j)>)

with a number of cross-references to lower levels (see fig. 2).

2.4 Level 3: CASE (CA)

A case is the total of examinations and treatments of a patient performed by a single person or a group of persons within a

specific institution of the health care delivery system and it is
an episode as defined in |9|. The identifier, composed of place of
treatment and treating person is called health coordinate (HC).
Structure of level 3:

CA(HC, <LP(3i)>, <PL(3j)>, <EV(k)>).

2.5 Level 4: EVENT (EV)

On this level all data are aggregated which result from a meeting
of physician and patient. This data may be descriptions of the
system "patient" or interventions in parts of the patient's body or
functions. An event is unambiguously identified by patient
identification (level 1), association to a problem (level 2),
health coordinate (level 3) and date (level 4). This concept has
some analogy to COLLEN's "visit-oriented" basic structure |5|.
Structure of level 4:

EV(T(date), <LP(4i)>, <SO(j)>, <SI(k)>).

<SO(j)> is the list of system observations SO(j) (see chapter
2.6.1), <SI(k)> the list of system interventions SI(k) (see chapter
2.6.2).

2.6 Level 5: ACTIVITY

- System observation (SO)
- System intervention (SI)

The current detailed medical information which is produced by
system observing or intervening activities, is localized on this
lowest structural level.
Structure of level 5:

SO respect. SI(T(date), T(time), <SP(i...) (<<DF(i...d),
V(i...d)>>)>).

Qualified by the temporal coordinates "date of measure" and "time
of measure" the relevant sub-procedures SP(i...) associated with
each SO and SI of level 4 are specified on this level. The SP(i...)
are completed by the respective list of ordered pairs (or tupels)
<DF(i...d), V(i...)>, i.e. by the data formats used and the
corresponding results.

2.6.1 System observations

The system observations comprise all medical activities which are
performed to describe the past and/or present status of the system
"patient", namely symptoms (patient's statements), signs (doctor's
statements as results of examinations), tests and diagnostic
radiology.

The complete set of system observations SO(i) is described in a
procedure file which contains a number of specifications for each
SO(i).

The results of the various system observations which are stored in
the historical part of the CDB, are interpreted via the procedure
file, i.e. system-controlled and not through the logic of a
specific application program.

Further aspects which have to be analyzed more thoroughly are the extension of the procedure file to a general reference system for attribute-oriented queries and its incorporation into the data description part of the MANAGER.

2.6.2 System interventions

The notion "system interventions" covers all diagnostic and therapeutical measures which modify the system "patient" in any way. The catalogue of system interventions, which is managed by the procedure file as well, comprises the following procedures:

- Surgical procedures, anaesthetics, radiotherapy, physical therapy, drug therapy, psychotherapy, intensive care, haemodialysis.

Therapeutical procedures generally result in new patient system observations which again cause further intervening acts etc. Reichertz |8| generally analyzed the modes of proceeding in medicine and represented them by a cybernetic cycle:

signal production --> apperception --> interpretation --> act --> signal production....

A consequent acquisition of these interrelations results in recursive data structures which will be the basis of a therapy model. In the initial phase of the project this "feedback-loop" will mostly be left open, because of the lack of such therapy models. However, information linking the elements of the cybernetic cycle can be included in more or less formalized and structured form in the list of notes on level 4 thus providing for a data micro-structure with network relationships on the lower levels.

2.7 Data base descriptions

Fig. 2 shows the graph representation of the data structure model of the regional data base.

For the description of a data base the different approaches published up to now define several levels. The ANSI/X3/SPARC-Group |3| proposed a 3-schema-model:

- The "Conceptual Schema" describes those aspects of real objects on which data is stored in the data base and as data is viewed by the (non-programmer) user of the information system. In terms of HIS those "real objects" are the patients.

- The "External Schema" describes the data as it is viewed by the programmer, the so-called logical view.

- The "Internal Schema" describes the data as it is stored and handled by the data base system.

In terms of this approach the proposed data structure model is mainly representing the conceptual level yet comprising some elements of the external or logical and the internal or physical level, e.g. the hierarchical pointers.

To be useful as reference structure the model has to represent a global non-redundant view of the relevant slice of reality. A comprehensive conceptual model should include semantic information on objects and their relationships as well. This becomes especially

important for the correct use of inquiry systems which are at the
non-programmer's disposal. In this context the current research
activities on semantic networks and conceptual graphs to support a
natural language interface to data bases should be mentioned.

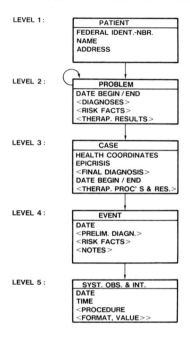

LEVEL 1:
| PATIENT |
| FEDERAL IDENT.-NBR. |
| NAME |
| ADDRESS |

LEVEL 2:
| PROBLEM |
| DATE BEGIN / END |
| <DIAGNOSES> |
| <RISK FACTS> |
| <THERAP. RESULTS> |

LEVEL 3:
| CASE |
| HEALTH COORDINATES |
| EPICRISIS |
| <FINAL DIAGNOSIS> |
| DATE BEGIN / END |
| <THERAP. PROC' S & RES.> |

LEVEL 4:
| EVENT |
| DATE |
| <PRELIM. DIAGN.> |
| <RISK FACTS> |
| <NOTES> |

LEVEL 5:
| SYST. OBS. & INT. |
| DATE |
| TIME |
| <PROCEDURE |
| <FORMAT, VALUE>> |

Fig. 2: The macro-structure of the conceptual HIS data structure
        model.

2.8 Data manipulation procedures

The data structure model of the health information system is
completed by a set of descriptions for all data manipulations resp.
transactions, the so-called <u>data</u> <u>manipulation</u> <u>procedures</u> |11|.

3. THE CONCEPT OF THE HIS DATA MANAGER

3.1 Tasks

The frequent changes in the structures of the data base as
mentioned in the introductory chapter, led to the development of a
data managing system for solving the following tasks |6|:

a. Provision for an automated documentation of the data structure
   model, and assist the system programmer with information about
   the most up-to-date version of that structure model.
b. In order to facilitate user programming the necessary
   accessing routines for the data manipulation language will be
   automatically generated.

c. A simple updating capability to modify and eventually generate the data structure model during the development phase and to satisfy future needs. Different versions of the structure model could be held under different names.

d. Communication with the Data Definition Language (DDL) of the Data Base Management System (DBMS) in use will be handled by an interface package.

e. A capability for simulation of search strategies in the data base.

f. A capability for estimation of the search times of the various data base accesses.

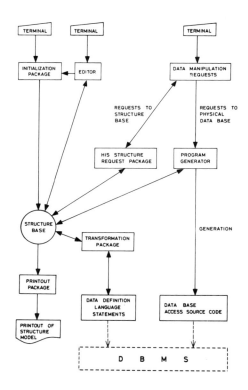

Fig. 3: Environment of the HIS data manager |6|.

3.2 HIS data manager functions

a. The MANAGER has its own description of the data structure model in a data base called the STRUCTURE BASE. The structure base is more detailed and commented than the Data Definition Language used by the Data Base Management System and allows for mapping between different structure models.

b. The content of the STRUCTURE BASE is automatically printable and thus serves directly as documentation of the data base.

c. The STRUCTURE BASE is interactively initialized.
d. Since some changes in the STRUCTURE BASE are not allowed an editor will check the legality of each modification and special attention is paid to the correctness of the secondary changes in the STRUCTURE BASE.
e. An DDL INTERFACE module contains transformation programs to transform the detailed STRUCTURE BASE contents into terms of the Data Definition Language used by the Data Base Management System and vice versa.
f. The Program Generator module generates source code (procedures) to do the data base accesses needed in the application programs. These accesses refer in terms of the Data Manipulation Language (DML) used by the Data Base Management System to elements of its structure descriptions.
g. The language in which the selection rules are formulated (request language) may have a structure similar to the Relational-Data-Base sublanguages, like for example Chamberlin's et.al. SEQUEL |4|. This request language should be highly interactive. It is based on a data structure which is very near to the conceptual structure model discussed in chapter 2 and which contains application-specific data types such as date or time.

The DATA MANAGER system concept is shown in fig. 3.

4. CONCLUSION

In this contribution the basic structure for the historical part of the Common Data Base of the Health Information System of Berlin is described. One of the main working objectives for the next future is the refinement of this basic structure.

It should be pointed out that this data structure is a conceptual working model representing the patient-oriented nucleus of the information system. In the course of developing HIS new information entities and other relationships between data, like those which are covered by the basic structure, will be introduced. Thus the hierarchical model will be extended to a more general graph model where some of the so-called "local properties" themselves - e.g. the health coordinates - will be associated with describing attributes or local properties and will therefore be expressed by relationship to new entities.

REFERENCES

| 1| Anonym: Abgeordnetenhaus von Berlin, Vorlage ueber die erste Fortschreibung des Berichts ueber die weitergehende Planung zur Automatisierung im Gesundheitswesen, Drucksache 6/977 vom 3.8.1973 Kulturbuchverlag, Berlin.
| 2| Anonym: Medizinisches Informationssystem, DOMINIG - Teilprojekt 1: Regionales medizinisches Organisations- und Planungssystem fuer ueberbetriebliche Aufgaben des oeffentlichen Gesundheitswesens, Senator fuer Gesundheit und Umweltschutz, Berlin, Nov. 1973.
| 3| ANSI/X3/SPARC, Study Group on Data Base Management Systems, Interim Report (Washington, DC: CBEMA 1975).
| 4| Boyce, Chamberlin, King III and Hammer: Specifying Queries as Relational Expressions, in Klimbie, Koffeman (Eds.): Data Base Management, IFIP Working Conference on Data Base Management, April 1974 (North-Holland, Amsterdam, 1974).

| 5| M.F. Collen, L.S. Davis and E.E. van Brunt: The Computer Medical Record in Health Screening, Meth. Inform. Med. 10 (1971) 138-142.

| 6| M. Jainz and T. Risch (Eds.): A Data-Manager for a Health Information System, Comp. Progr. Biomed. 6 (1976) 166-170.

| 7| V. Kaestner: The Development of a Computer Based Medical Information Support System for Berlin, Proceedings of MEDIS'73, Osaka, Japan.

| 8| P.L. Reichertz: Medizinische Informatik - Aufgabe, Wege und Bedeutung, Verh. Ges. Dtsch. Naturf. und Aerzte 1972, (Springer Verlag, Heidelberg, 1973) 106-120.

| 9| P.L. Reichertz: Datenbanken und Informationssysteme, in: S. Koller and G. Wagner (Eds.): Handbuch der medizinischen Dokumentation und Datenverarbeitung, (Schattauer, Stuttgart, 1975).

|10| K. Sauter, P.L. Reichertz and W. Zowe: Die zentrale Patienten-Datenbank in einem integrierten Hospitalinformationssystem, Meth. Inform. Med. 11 (1972) 91-96.

|11| K. Sauter (Ed.): A Data Structure Model for a Health Information System, Comp. Progr. Biomed. 6 (1976) 171-177.

|12| W. Schneider: Integration of Data from a Computer Automated Laboratory into a Generalized Hospital Information System, in: G. Griesser and G. Wagner (Eds.): Automatisierung des Klinischen Labors (Schattauer Verlag, Stuttgart-New York, 1968) 301-305.

|13| W. Schneider and S. Bengtsson (Eds.): The Application of Computer Techniques in Health Care, Comp. Prog. Biomed. 5 (1975) 169-250.

|14| L.L. Weed: Medical Records, Medical Education and Patient Care, Press of Case Western University, 1969.

Computational Linguistics in Medicine, Schneider/Sägvall Hein, eds.
North-Holland Publishing Company, (1977)

PSYPAC: A FORMAL SYSTEM FOR THE MODELLING OF COGNITIVE PROCESSES

R. Pfeifer and W. Schneider
Interdisziplinäre Konfliktforschungsstelle, University of Zürich
and
Uppsala University Data Center

in collaboration with
U. Moser and I. v. Zeppelin
Institute of Psychology, University of Zürich

PSYPAC is intended to be an instrument for building models of cognitive
processes in human behavior. It provides - in a very general sense - a
formalism for the description of such processes. An overview of the
structure and dynamics of the class of models that can be constructed
with PSYPAC is presented, as well as the set of primitives provided
allowing for easy model construction.

INTRODUCTION

PSYPAC is intended to be an instrument for building models of cognitive processes
in human behavior; it provides - in a very general sense - a formalism for the
description of such processes. A set of primitives is provided that allow for
easy specification of psychological entities and processes involved in a specific
model. A clear distinction between the PSYPAC level (also called the system
level) and the model level (of the model built with the PSYPAC system) will be
advocated throughout the paper.
Sections 1 and 2 present an outline of the class of models that can be constructed
as determined by the structure of PSYPAC, while section 3 describes what means
and aids are at disposition for the user to build his particular model. A specific
problem concerning implementation is brought up in section 4.

1. Structure of PSYPAC Models

A model built with PSYPAC consists of five major components: a PRIMARY ELEMENT
POOL, a TASK POOL, a TASK EXECUTOR, a MONITOR and a CONTROLLER.
All these components are defined upon the common basic notion of ELEMENT. The
structure of PSYPAC models should account for most of the cognitive processes
described in psychological literature.

1.1 ELEMENTs

ELEMENTs are hypothetical entities that cluster together certain types of information (1). We call our entities ELEMENTs to emphasize that they differ considerably
in some respects from existing notions such as "frames" (2) or "schemata" (3) although they do have much in common.
An ELEMENT consists of a PATTERN, ASSOCIATIONs and MANIPULATION SCHEMES as visua-
lized in Fig. 1.

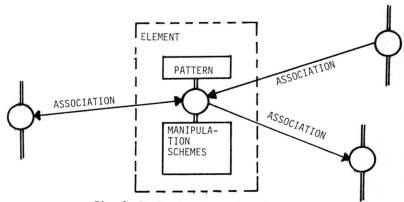

Fig. 1: Basic structure of an ELEMENT

1.1.1 PATTERNs

A PATTERN consists of a variety of information providing for a variety of ways to access an ELEMENT. It is an abbreviated coding of the contents of an ELEMENT e.g. in the form of an affective subpattern described in psychology. The functional significance of PATTERNs lies in their use by other model components as guiding cues for global quick search processes. The complete PATTERN uniquely identifies an ELEMENT. In general, however, only a part of the PATTERN is used during model operation (see section 2).

1.1.2 ASSOCIATIONs

ELEMENTs can be connected - for what reason ever - by establishing so called ASSOCIATIONs. For example it might be useful to tie one ELEMENT to another which is frequently referenced by it. ELEMENTs connected by ASSOCIATIONs can be viewed as having a high logical proximity even though there may be no or very little resemblance in the internal structure of the ELEMENTs. Functionally they serve "local" search mechanisms.

PSYPAC provides for a number of specific ASSOCIATIONs. An important one is "ISA", as defined by WINOGRAD (4), i.e. a connection of an ELEMENT to another from which it inherits properties unless specified differently.

1.1.3 MANIPULATION SCHEMES

MANIPULATION SCHEMES (we will use MS for MANIPULATION SCHEME in the sequel) are composits of explicit or implicit instructions involving referencing of other ELEMENTs. Unlike ASSOCIATIONs that are -so to speak - "wired" connections, they are open for different references to be established according to the CONTEXT (see below).

MSs have a unique name within the ELEMENT which has information attached to it either in the form of an executable procedure or in a way that a process for acquiring the information beeing looked for has to be set up first. The distinction is taken care of by those ELEMENTs which enclose ELEMENT evaluation procedures To locally direct operation of model components there is a special MS called SEQUENCE, namely a suggestion for the sequence in which to apply MSs if no other information is available. Another means of directing computation locally is by specifying ANTE and POST information within a MS. ANTE information is a list of possibilities that can be used before the reference is established, POST suggests what could be done after the reference has been established.

The notion of MSs resembles in some respect what WINOGRAD (4), calls IMPs (important elements).

There are two MSs of special importance, EXECUTE and REALIZE.

EXECUTE provides for a "look ahead" mechanism that can be useful in planning activities and accounts for internal (covert) tentative acting, a simulation of
possible effects. Depending on the references established by MSs EXECUTE contains
information concerning possible consequences, results, changes in the environment,
effort that would have to be put into the realization of the ELEMENT, ELEMENTs
that are likely to follow the present one, anticipated affect experiences etc..
Of course, look ahead information may in special cases also be provided by appropriate user defined MSs.
In a similar way, model dynamics require the introduction of a MS REALIZE used
for modelling actual physical behavior. REALIZE information corresponds to behavioral code which is loaded and executed involving the use of a preprocessor
system (see e.g. (5), (6), (7)). During REALIZATION of an ELEMENT actual changes
in the environment take place and the environment in turn can influence further
REALIZATION and further operation of the model in general.

1.1.4 Linguistic and non-linguistic processes

Many of the cognitive processes described in psychological literature are - at
least in part - of a non-linguistic nature such as the whole range of emotions
which are extremely important in human behavior. Thus the components of a model
must allow for description of such phenomena. An important area of future research is therefore the analysis of the interaction between these non-linguistic
phenomena (such as defence processes in the theory of neurosis) and linguistic
behavior.
Linguistic references can be modelled by using the COG-NAME feature which is part
of the recognition PATTERN of an ELEMENT. Other subpatterns (e.g. perceptual or
affective) are used in addition for determining the CONTEXT (see paragraph 2.3).
Note that several ELEMENTs can have the same COG-NAME subpattern.
In a text understanding TASK (definition of TASKs, see paragraph 1.2.2) it may be
the case that an individual is not capable of catching the correct meaning even
though all corresponding ELEMENTs have been defined. The reason for this could be
that via the COG-NAME subpattern a reference to an inaccessible ELEMENT is tried
to be established. Inaccessible signifies that the ELEMENT has to be avoided by
means of defence mechanisms because e.g. too much anxiety would be aroused by
accessing the ELEMENT. In such a case it is, of course, impossible for the individual to get the correct reading of the text.
We believe that the availability of the COG-NAME feature is one step in the
direction of investigating the interaction between the two different kinds of
processes. For problems of communication, i.e. to generate discourse, a verbalization routine is attached which in the case of ELEMENTs having a COG-NAME may be a
procedure which simply returns the COG-NAME subpattern. For ELEMENTs without a
COG-NAME subpattern, the routine is more complex. The feasibility of introducing
a set of general verbalization routines (e.g. for the description of certain
TYPEs of ELEMENTs without a COG-NAME) is under investigation.
The notion of a COG-NAME has to be distinguished from the case when the modeller
- for the purpose of communication - names certain ELEMENTs even if they do not
have a COG-NAME (e.g. a defence mechanism); the ELEMENT is then said to have a
MODEL-NAME. The MODEL-NAME is attached to the PATTERN of an ELEMENT as an artificial subpattern with no functional significance whatsoever (see also section 3).

1.2 Model Components

1.2.1 PRIMARY ELEMENT POOL

PRIMARY ELEMENTs (we will use PE for PRIMARY ELEMENT in the sequel) are the basic
domain specific constituents of a PSYPAC model on which other model components
operate. The recognition PATTERN of a PE contains information which classifies it
as belonging to the PRIMARY ELEMENT POOL.
The application of PSYPAC to actual modelling projects shows that the definition
of model specific TYPEs of PEs is necessary for the modelling process. The TYPE
information is entered as part of the PATTERN. For the purpose of illustration let
us just briefly comment on two examples, PEs of TYPE ACTION-ELEMENT and ABSTRACT-

ELEMENT (see Fig. 2). ACTION-ELEMENTs are PEs that can potentially be executed

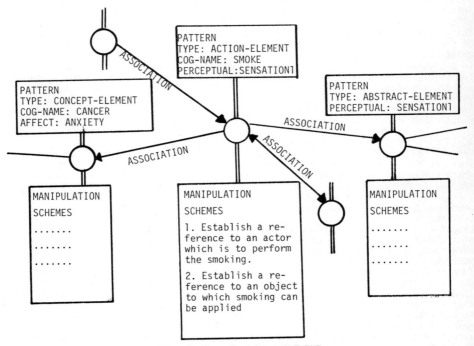

Fig. 2: Example of an ELEMENT

and realized. Frequently they have as their COG-NAME subpattern a verb. ABSTRACT-ELEMENTs are used in connection with ACTION-ELEMENTs. They are constructs showing preferred ways of performing the corresponding ACTION-ELEMENTs. Note that in general an ABSTRACT-ELEMENT does not have a COG-NAME subpattern.
The decision concerning the choice of types to be introduced should be made by the modeller of a particular application since the optimum choice may vary from domain to domain.

1.2.2 TASK POOL
The TASK POOL is a set of ELEMENTs, called TASKs (8), i.e. ELEMENTs that demand action from the TASK EXECUTOR described in the next paragraph. They are the basic units that trigger the dynamic operation of the model. TASKs can be activated by different processes: by an intrinsic motivational system, by input from the outside world into the model, or by beeing generated and invoked by the TASK EXECUTOR or the CONTROLLER.

1.2.3 The TASK EXECUTOR
The TASK EXECUTOR (8) is an active component of the model, a set of ELEMENTs for performing TASKs in accordance to the information comprised in their PATTERNs, ASSOCIATIONs and MSs. It strongly interacts with the MONITOR and the CONTROLLER.

1.2.4 The MONITOR
The MONITOR (8) is also an active component of the model in charge of signalling

to the CONTROLLER (see next paragraph) whenever a situation arises that questions further smooth operation of the model. It signals deviations of parameters from a predefined range (especially important for affective processes). This includes checking the resource utilization (e.g. if a process demands resources currently not available from an external source).
Briefly the MONITOR performs a large number of tests and generates interrupts and messages for further processing by the CONTROLLER.

1.2.5 The CONTROLLER
A third active component of a PSYPAC model is the CONTROLLER (8) which is in charge of maintaining smooth operation of the model. It analyzes conditions communicated by the MONITOR and generates and schedules processes that bring the model parameters back into a normal range.
The interaction of the CONTROLLER, the MONITOR and the TASK EXECUTOR can he described by the following example. Assume an individual is involved in a problem solving TASK. The TASK EXECUTOR generates as one of its subtasks a TASK which implies a matching process. For some reason, e.g. from experience, anxiety is beeing generated through activation of a certain ELEMENT. If the anxiety level deviates too much from given limits the MONITOR signals this exceptional condition to the CONTROLLER, which in turn has to decide what processes to start to achieve regular conditions again. One possibility is to stop this particular activity, chunking some of the information together into a TASK and putting it into a "deferred store" for later processing.
This can, of course, severely interfere with the current problem solving behavior. The example just described is typical for situations occurring in the course of a dream.

2. Dynamics of PSYPAC models
In this section a few PSYPAC facilities that account for the required dynamics of psychological models are briefly described.

2.1 Activation of Model Operation
In order to activate model operation there must be driving forces. PSYPAC models can either be
(a) input driven: processing is triggered by information from the environment (language, feedback information from physical behavior in the REALIZE mode etc.). As input we consider all information reaching the cognitive system through a preprocessor system (see also paragraph 1.1.3),
(b) driven by intrinsic motivational processes: for some reason a cognitive ELEMENT is activated and processing continues from this ELEMENT with or without any interaction with the environment, or
(c) driven by model operation itself: during the course of TASK performance new TASKs can be generated as subtasks or as TASKs to be performed during or after completion of the current one.
By these three mechanisms TASKs can be added to the TASK POOL for performance by the TASK EXECUTOR, which in turn has to be able to process ELEMENTs. This is provided for by a number of special evaluation mechanisms described in the next paragraph.

2.2 Evaluation of ELEMENTs
Each part of an ELEMENT is processed in a different mode.

Evaluation of a PATTERN
Only the PATTERN of the ELEMENT is inspected and no look "into" the ELEMENT is performed. This is the most superficial but also the fastest type of processing. The result is a general idea of what the ELEMENT is about. This mode of evaluation can be applied to all ELEMENTs since all have (by definition) a PATTERN. It is of great importance for the description of psychic processes that proceed by only inspecting affect subpatterns.
Most commonly this processing mode is used for matching a given PATTERN or sub-

pattern against other ones. This mechanism provides a means for quick search processes over a large number of ELEMENTs. Processing of the PATTERN only is also
used in the simulation of a resonance retrieval principle: get all ELEMENTs which
have a common subpattern. This is accomplished by a special type of MS, REVERBE-
RATE. The introduction of a resonance retrieval principle requires an inhibition
mechanism which is invoked under conditions to be defined by the user (see also
9).

Evaluation of ASSOCIATIONs

This mechanism simply traces ASSOCIATIONs and returns the associated ELEMENTs. It
can be viewed as a local kind of search mechanism. Although the ASSOCIATION information can be processed separately it is commonly used in connection with MSs
to be applied e.g. as a first guess (see below).

Evaluation of MANIPULATION SCHEMES

One or more MSs of an ELEMENT can be applied according to the current needs of
model operation. Here the local information given in SEQUENCE (special MS, see
paragraph 1.1.3) and within an MS the ANTE and POST information can be used or
overriden as described earlier. These mechanisms may take advantage of ASSOCIA-
TIONs.

Only two MSs, EXECUTE and REALIZE, are discussed here in more detail. Evaluation
of an EXECUTE MS (also called executing an ELEMENT) corresponds to looking ahead
in the planning process. Before an ELEMENT can be executed the relevant references to other ELEMENTs have to be established: In the example of Fig. 2 the reference to the smoker (e.g. the individual John) and the reference to the object to
be smoked (e.g. a cigarette). In this way a number of possible consequences can
be determined depending on the CONTEXT.

Evaluation of a REALIZE MS (also called realizing an ELEMENT) signifies that the
routines for performing actual physical behaviour are loaded and executed.
A precondition is, as in the case of EXECUTE that the relevant references have
been established. Realizing an ELEMENT induces changes in the external world
(anticipated or unexpected). These processes return feedback information from the
environment to be used in further processing. This leads to a complex interaction
between the planning process (and possibly other cognitive activities) and the
realization process.

2.3 CONTEXT

All processing during model operation takes place within a so called CONTEXT. We
use an implicit notion of CONTEXT. It is determined by the current state of the
model (CONTROLLER, MONITOR, TASK EXECUTOR and the set of activated TASKs and PEs
at a given time).

2.4 Creating New ELEMENTs and ASSOCIATIONs

During model operation new ELEMENTs can be created. The different active model
components must comprise a number of mechanisms that allow for dynamic creation
of new ELEMENTs. Psychological literature suggests many kinds of cognitive activities in which new ELEMENTs are generated. Furthermore there must be mechanisms
for establishing new ASSOCIATIONs during model operation.

3. Modelling Aids

For the class of possible models described in sections 1 and 2 PSYPAC contains
modelling aids. They provide for easy model construction. PSYPAC comprises the
following modelling aids: primitives for definition of the earlier described
model components, a print package that allows for printing ELEMENTs, and for
tracing model activities during operation etc., a set of administration primitives (file handling, documentation etc.), a set of general purpose functions that
can be used in hand-coding, and a set of primitives to describe specific linguistic processes.

Since a lengthy discussion of the details is beyond the scope of this paper, we
will just comment on one example, the definition of ELEMENTs: For technical rea-

sons the PSYPAC system tends to transform PATTERNs and subpatterns into an internal representation. As long as the system does not have to communicate it will work with this representation as far as possible. The modeller has the choice to work in any representation he desires, i.e. via COG-NAMEs only, via a number of subpatterns, via a MODEL-NAME (which he can choose to attach to the PATTERN of an ELEMENT for the purpose of communication with the system, but which does not participate in model activities) or directly via the internal representation. Working on the internal representation prevents disambiguation processes but is not very comfortable. Working on COG-NAMEs only is easier but might lead to a number of additional questions asked by the system to be sure of the intended meaning of the modeller. If, e.g. one wishes to define ASSOCIATIONs between ELEMENTs, PATTERNs, any representation can be used. If ambiguities occur an interactive disambiguation routine is called. If references to non-existing ELEMENTs are to be established, a message is printed and the non-existing ELEMENT is put on a waiting list for later definition. ELEMENTs on the waiting list are also taken into account when establishing further ASSOCIATIONs. The same holds for the introduction of undefined ELEMENTs while defining MSs. The system is able to run models that are incompletely defined. On encountering an undefined ELEMENT during model operation the system will print a message. Furthermore, if an item (any kind of expression) is encountered which does not conform to PSYPAC syntax, a message is printed that the item cannot be handled by standard PSYPAC supported functions (except for very superficial kinds of manipulation). Non-standard information can be introduced by the user but he then must himself take care that this information is processed correctly. If the model encounters either an undefined ELEMENT or a non-standard item, after printing a message, operation is tried to be continued. If an undefined ELEMENT has to be processed (if it does not have to be processed this is irrelevant to model operation), a further MS is beeing tried e.g., to find another suitable ELEMENT.
Only if all information on how to continue is exhausted, model operation is terminated.

4. A Remark on The Implementation of PSYPAC
The question arises what computer language should be used for the implementation of PSYPAC. Conventional programming languages such as FORTRAN, COBOL or PL1 are not taken into consideration because they do not provide a number of important facilities which are a prerequisite for an implementation. One of the few languages that actually fulfill the requirements is LISP. Of course, higher level AI (Artificial Intelligence) languages as e.g. MICRO-PLANNER (10), CONNIVER (11), QLISP (12), and also the recently developed KRL-0 (13) could be possible candidates. To some extent they would seem to be more suitable because they provide high level facilities such as e.g. pattern-matching and backtracking. They comprise, however, implicitly psychological hypotheses which induce an undesirable bias. The effort needed for eliminating this bias implies, however, that a straightforward implementation of PSYPAC in LISP is more adequate. Some of the high level facilities provided by other LISP based AI languages may easily be included in PSYPAC at a later stage. The reasons for choosing INTERLISP among the dialects of LISP were a "subset" of those summarized in (14), see (15).

References

(1a) R. Pfeifer, W. Schneider: PSYPAC: Internal report AD-G-03, Zürich and Uppsala, August, 1976.
(1b) R. Pfeifer: PSYPAC: Internal report AD-D-02, Zürich and Uppsala, April, 1977.
(2) M. Minsky: A Framework for Representing Knowledge. MIT AI Memo 306, 1974.
(3) D.G. Bobrow, D.A. Norman: Some Principles of Memory Schemata. In: D.G. Bobrow, A. Collins (Eds.): Representation and Understanding. New York: Academic Press, 1975, 131-149.
(4) T. Winograd: Frame Representations and the Declarative-Procedural Controversy. In: D.G. Bobrow, A. Collins (Eds.): Representation and Understandning. New York: Academic Press, 1975, 185-210.
(5) U. Moser, R. Pfeifer, W. Schneider, I. v. Zeppelin: Computersimulation von Schlaftraumprozessen. Schlussbericht an den Schweiz. Nat. Fonds, Nr. 1.434. 70, Zürich, 1976.
(6) E. Hunt: What Kind of Computer Is Man? Cognitive Psychology, 1971, 2, 57-98.
(7) E. Hunt: The Memory We Must Have. In: R.C. Schank, K.M. Colby (Eds.): Computer Models of Thought and Language. San Francisco: W.H. Freeman, 1973, 343-371.
(8a) R. Pfeifer, W. Schneider: PSYPAC: Internal report AD-G-02, Zürich and Uppsala, January, 1975.
(8b) R. Pfeifer: PSYPAC: Internal report AD-D-01, Zürich and Uppsala, August, 1975.
(9) M. Cunningham: Intelligence: Its Organization and Development. New York: Academic Press, 1972.
(10) J.G. Sussman, T. Winograd, E. Charniak: MICRO-PLANNER Reference Manual. MIT AI Memo 203A, 1971.
(11) D.V. Modermott, G.J. Sussman: The CONNIVER Reference Manual. MIT AI Memo 259, 1972.
(12) R. Reboh, E. Sacerdoti: A Preliminary QLISP Manual. SRI Project 8721, Stanford, 1973.
(13) D.G. Bobrow, T. Winograd: An Overview of KRL, A Knowledge Representation Language. Manuscript, 1976.
(14) E. Sandewall: Programming in An Interactive Environment: The LISP Experience. Linköping University, 1976.
(15) R. Pfeifer, W. Schneider: PSYPAC: Internal report AD-G-01, Zürich and Uppsala, February 1974.

Computational Linguistics in Medicine, Schneider/Sagvall Hein, eds.
North-Holland Publishing Company, (1977)

C O N D O R
Communication in Natural Language
with Dialogue Oriented Retrieval
Systems

N. Banerjee
Data and Information Systems Group
Application Software
SIEMENS AG, Munich

1. The General Goal of CONDOR

The goal of Project CONDOR is to develope a general purpose
system capable of automatically collecting, describing, retrieving and processing structured and unstructured information. Natural language should be the language of communication between the
system and its users.

For the realization of this goal components are needed for

- automatic initial processing of texts (optical scanner)

- automatic analysis of natural language

- automatic classification of texts

- interactive collection of formattable data

- checking the validity of interactively collected data

- storing primary data (i. e. texts and formatted fields)
  and secondary data (i. e. inverted files, document
  networks, semantic networks) in a data base

- accessing the data base by means of natural language

- accessing the data base by means of a formalized
  command language

- evaluating and processing the data stored in the data base

- aiding in planning and realizing control mechanisms for
  the communication between the system and its users

- generating individual systems from the available
  modular components so that the needs of individual
  users can be optimally met.

The greater part of these components exists presently as models.
A product version will be available in the early 1980's.

This project is supported by the German Federal Ministry of
Research and Technology.

163

2. Principles of CONDOR System Design

CONDOR aims at providing tools in the form of software components for processing all those kinds of information which are
encountered in information storage and retrieval applications.
These tools are being developed with certain principles in mind:

- the system must be able to manipulate both structured and
  unstructured information

- the software components developed must be highly adaptive

- the user must find communication with the system comfortable and easy

- the software components must be easy to maintain.

3. Manipulation of Structured and Unstructured Information

Applications in information storage and retrieval today require
the ability to process and access both structured and unstructured information. In the past, different systems have been used
for the two kinds of data. However, the needs of future users
require an integrated processing for both types, as the information sought will generally be a mixture of the two. For this
reason, CONDOR provides components for the integrated processing
of formatted and unformatted information. Such an integrated
system has the added advantage of being more economical and
easier to maintain than two separate systems.

4. Adaptive Programming

Our aim is to develope a system capable of learning on the basis
of the information it has access to. Learning means in this case
the ability to deduce metainformation by analysing different
characteristics of the information stored. General rules and
principles inherent in the information form the output of the
learning process. The system can then improve itself by using
this metainformation for future processing. Each software
component of CONDOR is being developed according to this
principle.

This way of constructing a system has several advantages, not
the least of which is that the necessity of manually/intellectu-
ally manipulating is reduced to a minimum. This is true for all
information processed, be it target information or secondary
information used to process and access the target information. A
consequence of this method is that an adaptive program will, in
the beginning, have less information and therefore produce
weaker output than a program which is not supposed to learn. A
rigid system of the non-learning type requires high quality and
manually prepared input for each application in order to be able
to produce a certain predetermined output. A learning system,
however, has a much wider range of applications and can, with
time, achieve an even better performance than a rigid non-learning system.

To elaborate this point I would like to describe two essential
components of CONDOR in some detail.

4.1. Natural Language Analysis

One component of CONDOR analyses natural language texts
syntactically and semantically. Generally, the first step in
automatic language analysis is to determine the syntactic function of each word in a sentence. In order to make this analysis
step possible, we proceeded in an unusual way. We did not start
by building up a lexicon containing a large number of significant words together with various kinds of grammatical information, such as parts of speech, conjugation, declination,
semantic markers etc. Instead, we built up a lexicon of function words containing about 800 entries (prepositions, pronouns,
articles, auxiliary verbs etc.) For the rest, i. e. for nouns,
adjectives, adverbs and verbs in all inflected forms, we
constructed an algorithm. This algorithm, the context-free
word analysis, was supplied with a limited number of
morphographematical rules, by means of which it ascertains the
syntactic function or functions each word can have. Since the
amount of metainformation, in this particular case morphographematical information, was small in the beginning, the
error rate was rather high. We kept on feeding the program
for each error with the corresponding correct result. The
program is so constructed that it can, on the basis of this
input, amend the rule, the metainformation, which caused the
error. In this way we have developed a word analysis algorithm,
which, applied to any German text, has an error rate of about
10 %. We are confident that the next version of this program,
which is now in preparation, will have an error rate of no
more than 2 %.

All other components of the natural language analyser are
constructed according to the same principle.

4.2. Automatic Classification of Texts

The natural language analyser has two different aims:

   a) to enable the user to put his·query in natural language,
      and
   b) to select key words or key phrases out of each
      document input to the data base.

The key words are then ranked using various statistical
operations. We have a ranking scale which is proportional to
the number of documents in the data base. For about 2000
documents the scale has 11 ranks, we call them "Prioritätsklas-
sen"; for about a million documents 20 ranks. The ranks can be
considered as horizontal layers of a pyramidal hierarchy.

Several programs using mathematical set operations and
statistical methods form at first a number of clusters of
terms within each rank. Other programs operate then on the
clusters across the ranks to interlink them. In this way we
obtain fully automatically a network of clusters, where each
cluster consists of a set of keywords. The relationship between the keywords of a cluster has been determined by
linguistic and statistical criteria. Since at the same time
every cluster represents a number of documents for which the
keywords of the cluster are typical, we obtain simultaneously

a classification of all the documents contained in the data
base. Our goal is to achieve a thematic classification of
these documents. This would mean that a data base containing,
for instance, documents in medicine, data processing and law
should be classified by this method into three groups and
each of these main groups into subclasses. If the data
processing documents dealt, for instance, with data terminal
and programming languages, and the latter documents again
could be subdivided into those dealing with machine-oriented
languages and those with problem-oriented languages, then
it should be possible using this method to obtain such a
classification automatically. We cannot claim to have reached
this ideal goal already, but the results obtained so far
are very satisfactory.

The aim of the classification is to achieve an optimal balance
between recall and precision: i. e. to include as many
relevant and to exclude as many irrelevant documents as
possible. This desired quality of the system can only be
achieved by making the classification programs   adaptive.
This again has a parallel in the developement of the natural
language analyser where the initial weak performance was
not to be avoided but is, in fact, being continually improved
by means of repeated learning.

The present performance of the system must be seen in
conjunction with the following points.

    The quality of the hierarchical classification is
    absolutely dependent on the quality of clusters, which
    again closely depends upon the reliability of the
    linguistic ranking criteria used to select the keywords
    and the statistical criteria used to form clusters by
    associating thematically related keywords and to
    interrelate the clusters. All these criteria contain a
    number of threshold values. It will be necessary to vary
    these threshold values by trial and error until an
    optimal balance is achieved. Our aim is to let the program
    do it on its own. We intend to conduct retrieval tests
    systematically and feed the program with the results
    and their corrections. This should then be the basis for
    the program to modify the threshold values until the
    clusters are properly regrouped and the interlinkage
    of the clusters is accordingly modified.

    We are experimenting at present with several data bases.
    These contain documents numbering between 200 and 2000.
    It is intended to increase the number to about 20,000 as
    soon as a series of retrieval tests on the present basis
    are completed.
    We always use a heterogeneous data base irrespective of
    the size. This means that even a small data base
    containing only 200 documents would be a mixture of
    medical, data processing, legal and miscellaneous
    newspaper texts. The system cannot therefore have
    sufficient vocabulary at its disposal for each subject.
    This causes a certain amount of instability, which can only
    be removed by expanding the data base. In spite of this
    fact the average precision rate at present is about 60 %.

The recall rate has not yet been worked out.

Finally, the performance of the natural language analyser
contributes significantly to the performance of the
classification system, and this analyser is not yet fully
developed. The present natural language analyser can
interprete the syntactic structure of a sentence. The
performance is quite satisfactory for our purposes,
although a few necessary components exist only in
rudimentary form. The semantic interpretation of natural
language statements will be realized gradually in the
near future. Under these circumstances it is obvious that
the linguistic ranking criteria used to select keywords
out of documents are not as powerful as they once will be.
This has naturally a direct impact on the quality of text
classification.

We are confident that system performance will be improved
significantly as soon as the problems discussed above are
gradually mastered.

4.3.   Adaptive Programming: More Generalised Programs
        and Wider Applicability

Using two important components of CONDOR as examples, I
have discussed some consequences of adaptive programming
in detail. I think it has been made clear that, although a
system designed primarily of learning algorithms will have a
weaker performance in the beginning, in the long run it will
have several advantages. One of these advantages, the reduction of the necessity to manipulate information manually/
intellectually, has already been discussed. The initial
intellectual investment for establishing the basic working
information is kept to a minimum while the programs are
constructed in such a way that they can "learn" from
corrected results.

Such generalised programs have a much wider range of
applicability than do rigid non-learning systems. For
instance,the natural language analyser can be used to analyse
any German sentence with relative accuracy although still a
model and not yet fully developed. What is more remarkable
is the fact that the same system can be used as basic software
for analysing other languages such as English, French etc!

5.   Easy Handling for System User

In order to achieve optimal acceptability it will be
necessary to provide users with outstanding facilities for
easy handling of the system. These facilities must cover
all user activities needed for collecting, describing,
retrieving and processing structured as well as unstructured
data.

5.1.   Data Collection

A constant bottleneck of almost all information systems
is data collection. This is due to the fact that the amount
of manual activity needed to collect data is, compared with

such activities needed to run and maintain a system,
extremely high. It is therefore necessery to do the utmost
to develope better facilities for collecting data.
Otherwise the usefulness of even very powerful automatic
information systems would be greatly impaired.

5.1.1. Optical Scanning of Original Documents

To solve at least a part of this problem we are developing
a system for optically scanning texts and diagrams of
original documents, such as books, newspapers, magazines.
This system combines a general font register with software
which enables the system to "learn" to read new kinds of type,
and software which provides feedback between the scanner and
certain programs of the natural language analyser to help
reduce the rate of scanning error. This system is already
in use.

5.1.2. Editing of Primary Information

Before documents can be input to a data base it is very often
necessary to edit the primary information. This editing can
include correcting, typing and printing mistakes or
modifying some part of the information for other reasons.
This job, especially the correction work, is very tedious and
time consuming. CONDOR will have utilities to facilitate
editing. For example it is possible in very many cases to
detect orthographic mistakes by means of digram and trigram
check routines. The rejected words and their context can
then be shown to the editor, allowing him to correct them
easily.

5.1.3. Describing Information Structures

A data base can hardly have any information which is totally
unstructured. Every text has at least a minimum of structure
if only in chapters, headings, subheadings etc. Most often
a document will be supplemented with additional information
such as author's name, publishing year etc. All these kinds
of information are required as search arguments while
retrieving. A powerful retrieval component must allow the
user considerable flexibility in building up his query
statements even if they refer, partly or wholly, to such
structured information. Such a reference should be possible
even if the user does not know under what label a particular
piece of information has been stored or what structural
relation it has to other units of information. Such
flexibility is only possible if the system has detailed
knowledge of all characteristics of these structural
relations. It should be possible to describe these
characteristics in terms of a set of attributes inherently
known to the system. It would however not suffice if the
description consisted alone of a declaration of the formats
of the fields and their labels. It will also be necessary
to describe the connotation, the properties and the
qualities of the content of the structure. Only then will
the user have the possibility of retrieving an object by
referring to it **indirectly, which** is a fundamental requirement
of a flexible retrieval dialogue.

A component of CONDOR called "das System der Strategischen Problembeschreibung" (System for the strategic description of problems and related objects) is being developed to make such a description of information structures possible. Actually it is being developed as a general purpose system for describing any kind of problem or object. In the first phase a problem is resolved into its constituent parts. The next step is the description of a set of attributes for each part so that its functions with respect to the whole or to other parts are defined. The ensuing results are contained in what we call a grammer, according to which, in a second phase, any object pertaining to this particular problem may be described. An advantage of such a system is the fact that all objects dealing with a particular problem are described in a similar way with similar vocabulary, leading ultimately to a classification of all objects described, in the sense that all objects having similar properties are clustered together.

5.2. Information Retrieval

So far, I have dealt with those components of CONDOR which are necessary for generating a data base. It might appear rather strange that, although the acronym CONDOR suggests that it is basically a dialogue system for communicating in natural language with data bases, so much effort is invested in developing software for generating a data base. This obvious discrepancy has a historical background. At the outset of this project we were of the opinion that, in order to ensure users flexible handling of an information retrieval system or a data base system, it would be sufficient to develope a highly sophisticated natural language analyser which could then act as a preprocessor to formalize user's search statements. We assumed that it would be possible to accomplish a noticeable increase in the overall performance of an information system by annexing such a preprocessor to the rest of the system without bothering about

a) the content and structure of the data base and

b) the retrieval strategy used to match the user's query with information stored in the system.

As work on the project proceeded, it became evident that such an approach would not lead to a satisfactory solution.

We came to the following conclusions:

- our system must coordinate the procedures for generating the data base with those for interpreting user's queries

- our system must serve as an intermediary between the user and the data base.

5.2.1. Coordination of Procedures for Generating the Data Base and for Interpreting User's Queries

Generating a data base always means, quite independent of the methods applied to do so, structuring and classifying the sum total of information to be included in the data base. If, however, the method used differs from the one used to interpret the search statement, then the result obtained by matching the outputs of both procedures, which is the output of the retrieval process, will generally be poor. This will be the case if on the one hand the user has the liberty to formulate his search statement freely and on the other the classification of the data base is achieved manually or even automatically, but using, for instance, only statistical operations, and not the natural language analyser used to interpret the freely formulated search statement.

We concluded therefore that if we allow users of our system to use natural language, and this we must if we want to offer him flexible handling, then we must use the same principles for generating the data base. It must be guaranteed that if the system simulates understanding natural language with respect to the user, then it must also do so with respect to its own data base.

5.2.2. Clarification Dialogue as Intermediary between User and Data Base

The CONDOR clarification dialogue operates on the basis of two different sources of information: the one coming from the user in the form of a search statement, analysed and structured by the natural language analyser, and the other from the data base in the form of a hierarchy of clusters of terms obtained by text classification (see 4.2.) or clusters of properties obtained by object classification (see 5.1.3.) A clarification dialogue becomes necessary if the very first matching of these two kinds of information does not result in a direct hit. In such a case the CONDOR clarification dialogue has the following possibilities.

5.2.2.1. Request User to Modify Query

The system may request the user to modify his query either by rephrasing a part or the whole of it or by volunteering additional information. Such a case may arise under two different circumstances.

a) The matching of the search arguments with the data base shows that the user's query is too general in the sense that it leads to the retrieval of too many documents out of too many different areas. This will be the case if e. g. all terms used in the query are located in the higher ranks (general terms) in the hierarchy of term clusters. In such a case it would be useful to ask the user to qualify some or all such terms to make his query more precise.

b) Some search arguments, which the linguistic analysis
of the query determines to be highly relevant, cannot
be identified by the system. In such a case it will
not be very economical to try to retrieve documents
on the basis of the remaining search arguments and
the system, recognizing this, requests the user to
give synonyms for these search arguments.

5.2.2.2. Guidance of User by Offering Information in the Data Base

If a user is searching for an object structured and
described with the help of the component "Strategische
Problembeschreibung" (see 5.1.3.), then it is possible to
offer a list of connotations which come close to the
properties of the object looked for. The user can then
choose those properties which he considers to be relevant.
This procedure can be repeated at each step of the
retrieval process, so that the necessary clarification of
the user's problem can be achieved under the guidance of
the system.

A similar procedure can be applied for the clarification
of a user's problem if he is searching for predominantly
unstructured textual documents. In this case the user is
guided by those parts of the term cluster hierarchy which
seem to have close affinity to his query.

6. Easy Maintenance of the System

The cost of maintaining complex systems must be reduced
drastically if manufacturers are to be able to continue
producing them. Such a reduction is also in the interest
of system users, especially when one considers the fact
that repairing information systems as they are today is
extremely time consuming. It causes an interruption in the
updating of the system, making it too unreliable for many
applications.

If the goal of having a system which is optimally easy to
maintain is to be achieved, it must be part of the design
strategy for each individual system component. One feature
of CONDOR contributing significantly to this goal, the
component for defining the logical sequences of control,
will be considered here. Our practice of adaptive
programming described earlier (see 4.) also simplifies
the maintenance problem to a great extent. Wherever this
method is applicable, it will no longer be necessary to
rewrite programs unless they need to be redesigned. It is
well known that the rewriting of a program brings new
errors. This vicious circle has a large share in the high
cost of maintenance.

6.1. Definition of Logical Sequences of Control

A major part of each program and program system is the
internal control sequence. We have developed a basic
control system that can be used interactively to define
any logical control sequence. The logical sequence of
control is stored in a control file and need not be coded.
Thus the share of program code in the whole system can
be reduced considerably. We intend to use this system not
only for programming each component but also for designing
future system versions. This will enable a high degree of
standardisation in designing and programming, which again
will make maintenance easier. For the same reason the
basic control system has been so constructed that it
supports the programmer in documenting what is produced
by demanding, while he is defining the logical sequence
of control, verbal and parametric information about the
function of each step defined. In other words, instead of
the usual post-documentation, which is dubious anyway,
the CONDOR system will have parallel documentation, which
records the intention of the programmer at a stage when
he still knows what he is doing, and which can be
regularly updated during each modification of the program.

LITERATURE

Anderson J R, Bower G H, Human Associative Memory, John Wiley, New York, 1973.

Bleich H L, The computer as a consultant, New England Journal of Medicine, vol. 284, pp 141-147, January 1971.

Bobrow D G, Collins A (eds.), Representation and Understanding, Academic Press, New York, 1975.

Bobrow D G, Winograd T, An overview of KRL, a knowledge representation language, Xerox Palo Alto Research Center Report, May 1976.

Bobrow D G, Raphael B, New programming languages for artificial intelligence research, Computing Surveys, vol. 6, no. 3, September 1974.

Brachman R J, What's in a Concept: Structural Foundations for Semantic Networks, BBN Report 3433, October 1976.

Brook R H, Williams K N, Avery A D, Quality assurance today and tomorrow: forecast for the future, Annals of Internal Medicine, vol. 85, pp 809-817, December 1976.

Bross, I D J, Shapiro P A, Anderson B B, How information is carried in scientific sublanguages, Science, vol. 176, pp 1303-1307, June 23, 1972.

Chalmers T C, A shortage of reliable data, New England Journal of Medicine, vol. 294, no. 14, pp 721-722, March 25, 1976.

Charniak E, Wilks Y (eds.), Computational Semantics, North-Holland Publishing Co., 1976.

Codd E, Seven steps to rendevous with the casual user, in Data Base Management, J W Klimbie & K I Koffeman (eds.), North-Holland Publishing Co., 1974.

Davis E, King J, An overview of production systems, Stanford University AI Memo 271, October 1975.

Davis R, Buchanan B, Shortliffe E H, Production rules as a representation for a knowledge-based consultation program, Artificial Intelligence, vol. 18, pp 15-45, 1977.

de Dombal F T, Grémy F (eds.), Decision Making and Medical Care: Can Information Science Help?, North-Holland Publishing Co., 1976.

Duda, R O, Hart P E, Nilsson N J, Subjective bayesian methods for rule based inference systems. Proc. 1976 National Computer Conference, vol. 45, pp 1075-1082, 1976.

Elstein A S, Clinical judgment: psychological research and medical practice, Science, vol. 194, pp 696-700, November 12, 1976.

Feinstein A, Clinical Judgment, Robert Krieger Publishing Company, Huntington, New York, 1967.

Fries J F, A data bank for the clinician, New England Journal of Medicine, vol. 294, no. 25, pp 1400-1402, June 17, 1976.

Fries J F, Alternatives in medical record formats, Medical Care, vol. 12, no. 10, pp 871-881, October 1974.

Groner G, Hopwood M, et al., An introduction to the Clinfo prototype data management and analysis system: release 2, Rand Report P-5617-1, February 1977.

Harless W G, Drennon G G, Maxer J J et al., Case: a natural language computer model, Computers in Biology and Medicine, vol. 3, pp 227-246, 1973.

Hirschman L, Grishman R, Sager N, From text to structured information: Automatic processing of medical reports, Proceedings of 1976 National Computer Conference, vol. 45, AFIPs Press, Montvale, New Jersey, pp 267-275, 1976.

Hoffer E P, Barnett G O, Farquhar B, Prather R A, Computer-aided instruction in medicine, in Annual Review of Biophysics and Bioengineering, vol. 4, L J Mullins (ed.), Annual Reviews Inc., Palo Alto, California, pp 103-118, 1975.

Hulse R K, Clark S J, Jackson J G, Werner H R, Gardner R M, Computerized medication monitoring system, American Journal of Hospital Pharmacy, vol. 33, pp 1061-1064, October 1976.

Kamp M, Index to Computerized Teaching in the Health Sciences, University of California, San Francisco, October 1975.

Kulikowski C A, Safir A, Concepts of computer-based modeling for consultation in optics and refraction, Proceedings 1976 ACM Conference, ACM, New York, pp 110-114, 1976.

Kulikowski C A, Weiss S, Trigboff M, Safir A, Clinical consultation and the representation of disease processes: some AI approaches, Rutgers University, Department of Computer Science Report CBM TR 58, January 1976.

Lindsay P H, Norman D A, Human Information Processing, Academic Press, 1975.

McDonald C J, Protocol-based computer reminders, the quality of care and the non-perfectability of man, New England Journal of Medicine, vol. 295, no. 24, pp 1351-1355, December 9, 1976.

Miller G A, Johnson-Laird P N, Language and Perception, Harvard University Press, Cambridge, Massachusetts, 1976.

Minsky M, A framework for representing knowledge, in The Psychology of Computer Vision, P Winston (ed.), McGraw-Hill, New York, pp 211-277, 1975.

Murphy E A, The Logic of Medicine, John Hopkins University Press, Baltimore, Maryland, 1976.

Newell A, Simon H A, Human Problem Solving, Prentice Hall, Englewood Cliffs, New Jersey, 1972.

Nilsson N J, Artificial Intelligence, Proceedings 1974 IFIP Conference, North-Holland Publishing Co., pp 778-801, 1974.

Norman D A, Rumelhart D E (eds.), Explorations in Cognition, W H Freeman, San Francisco, 1975.

Pauker S G, Gorry G A, Kassirer J P, Schwartz W B, Towards the simulation of clinical cognition: taking a present illness by computer, American Journal of Medicine, vol. 60, pp 931-996, 1976.

Pauker S G, Coronary artery surgery: the use of decision analysis, Annals of Internal Medicine, vol. 85, pp 8-18, 1976.

Palley N, Groner G, Sibley W, Hopwood M, Clinfo Users Guide: Release one, Rand Corporation Report R-1543-1, April 1976.

Petrick S, On natural language based computer systems, IBM Journal of Research and Development, pp 314-325, July 1976.

Pople H E, Myers J D, Miller R A, Dialog: a model of diagnostic logic for internal medicine, Proc. 4IJCAI, pp 848-855, 1975.

Pratt A W, Medicine, computers and linguistics, in Advances in Biomedical Engineering, vol. 3, Academic Press, New York, pp 97-140, 1973.

Rosati R, McNeer F, Starmer F, A new information system for medical practice, Archives of Internal Medicine, vol 135, pp 1017-1024, August 1975.

Rubin A, The role of hypotheses in medical diagnosis, Proc. 4IJCAI, pp 856-862, 1975.

Rychener M D, Production systems as a programming language for artificial intelligence applications, Technical Report Dept. of Computer Science, Carnegie-Mellon University, Pittsburgh, Pa., December 1976.

Sager N, Sublanguage grammars in science information processing, J. of the American Society for Information Science, vol. 26, no. 1, pp 10-16, 1975.

Schank R, Nash-Webber B L, Theoretical Issues in Natural Language Processing, Cambridge, Mass., June 1975.

Scott A C, Clancey W J, Davis R, Shortliffe E H, Explanation capabilities of production-based consultation systems, American Journal of Computational Linguistics, Microfiche 62, 1977.

Shortliffe E H, Computer Based Consultations: MYCIN, American Elsevier, New York, 1976.

Shortliffe E H, Buchanan B G, A model of inexact reasoning in medicine, Mathematical Biosciences, vol. 23, pp 351-379, 1975.

Starmer C, Rosati R, McNeer J, A comparison of frequency distributions for use in a model for selecting treatment in coronary artery disease, Computers in Biomedical Research, vol. 7, pp 278-293, 1974.

Susser M, Causal Thinking in the Health Sciences, Oxford University Press, New York, 1973.

Taylor T R, Clinical decision analysis, Methods of Information in Medicine, vol. 15, no. 4, pp 216-224, 1976.

Trigoboff M, Propagation of information in a semantic network, Proc. 1976 Artificial Intelligence & Simulation of Behavior Conference, Edinburgh, pp 334-343, 1976.

Tversky A, Kahneman D, Judgment under uncertainty: heuristics and biases, Science, vol. 185, pp 1124-1131, 1974.

Walker D E (ed.), Speech Understanding Research, Stanford Research Institute, Final Technical Report, October 1976.

Wechsler H, A fuzzy approach to medical diagnosis, Int. Journal of Bio-Medical Computing, vol. 7, pp 191-203, 1976.

Winston P H, Artificial Intelligence, Addison-Wesley, Reading, Massachusetts, 1977.

Wortman P H, Medical Diagnosis: an information processing approach, Computers in Biomedical Research, vol. 5, pp 315-328, 1972.

CONFERENCE COMMITTEES

Program committee

S Öhman	Uppsala University (Sweden)
A Pratt	NIH, Bethesda (USA)
A-L Sågvall Hein	UDAC, Uppsala (Sweden)
E Sandewall	University of Linköping (Sweden)
W Schneider, chairman	UDAC, Uppsala (Sweden)

Proceedings committee

A-L Sågvall Hein	UDAC, Uppsala
W Schneider	UDAC, Uppsala

Organizing committee

U Hein	UDAC, Uppsala
A-L Sågvall Hein, chairman	UDAC, Uppsala
W Schneider, v chairman	UDAC, Uppsala
K Sjöberg, secretary	UDAC, Uppsala

N. Banerjee
Siemens AG, Zentralbereich
Betriebswirtschaft
D-8000 München 70
Postfach 700070, F.R.G.

Stellan Bengtsson
Inst. f. Klin. Bakteriologi
Box 552
S-751 22 Uppsala
SWEDEN

Bernt Castman
Kommundata AB
Fack
S-126 12 Stockholm
SWEDEN

Carl Cederlund
IBM Medical Industry Center
Box 23006
S-104 35 Stockholm
SWEDEN

Michel de Heaulme
Faculté de Médecine
Pitié-Salpetrière
Dept. Biophys. et de Biomath.
91, Boulevard de l'Hopital
75634 Paris Cedex 13
FRANCE

Martin Epstein
Section on Medical Inf. Sci., Room A16
University of California
San Fransisco, California 94143
U.S.A.

Francois Grémy
Faculté de Médecine
Pitié-Salpetrière
Dept de Biophys. et de Biomath.
91, Boulevard de l'Hopital
75634 Paris Cedex 13
FRANCE

Gerd Griesser
Inst. f. Med. Stat. u. Dok.
2300 Kiel 1
Brunswiker Strasse 2 a
F.R.G.

Torgny Groth
UDAC, Box 2103
S-750 02 Uppsala
SWEDEN

Anders Grönwall
Akademiska sjukhuset
S-750 14 Uppsala
SWEDEN

Uwe Hein
UDAC, Box 2103
S-750 02 Uppsala
SWEDEN

Baldwin G. Lamson
Office of the Director
Hospitals and Clinics
The Center for Health Sciences, UCLA
Los Angeles, California 90024
U.S.A.

Lennart Naroskin
IBM Medical Industry Center
Box 23006
S-104 35 Stockholm
SWEDEN

Ruby Okubo
The Center for Health Sciences
UCLA, Los Angeles
California 90024
U.S.A.

Stephen G. Pauker
Department of Medicine
Tufts University School of Medicine
New England Medical Center
Boston, Massachusetts 02111
U.S.A.

Hans Peterson
Stockholms läns landsting
Centrala förvaltningen
Organisationsavdelningen
S-102 70 Stockholm
SWEDEN

Rolf Pfeifer
Soziologisches Institut der
Universität Zürich
Konfliktsforschungsstelle
Wiesenstrasse 9, 8008 Zürich
SWITZERLAND

Jan Pontén
Patologiska Institutionen
Dag Hammarskjölds väg 17
S-752 37 Uppsala
SWEDEN

Arnold W. Pratt
Div. of Computer Res. and Technology
Dept of Health, Education and Welfare
Bldg 12A, room 3033
NIH, Bethesda, Maryland 20014
U.S.A.

Hans-Åke Ramdén
UDAC, Box 2103
S-750 02 Uppsala
SWEDEN

Jan Roukens
SAZZOG Foundation
G.A. van Nispenstraat 37
Arnhem
THE NETHERLANDS

Anna-Lena Sågvall Hein
UDAC, Box 2103
S-750 02 Uppsala
SWEDEN

Erik Sandewall
Ämnesgruppen för datalogi
Matematiska Institutionen
Linköpings Universitet
S-581 83 Linköping
SWEDEN

Karl Sauter
Medizinische Hochschule Hannover
Dept Biometrie u. Med. Inf.
3 Hannover 61
Postfach 610180
F.R.G.

Werner Schneider
UDAC, Box 2103
S-750 02 Uppsala
SWEDEN

Edward H. Shortliffe
The MYCIN Project, Room TC110
Div. of. Clin Pharm.
Stanford Univ., School of Med.
Stanford, Cal. 94305
U.S.A.

William A. Spencer
Texas Institute for
Rehabilitation and Research
Texas Medical Center
P.O. Box 20095, Houston
Texas 77025, U.S.A.

Inga-Britt Sundin
Akademiska Sjukhuset
S-750 14 Uppsala
SWEDEN

Donna Taeuber
Siemens AG, Zentralbereich
Betriebswirtschaft
D-8000 München 70
Postfach 700070
F.R.G.

Jaak Urmi
Ämnesgruppen för Datalogi
Linköpings Universitet
S-581 83 Linköping
SWEDEN

Jan van Egmond
Medical Informatics Gent
Academic Hospital
135, De Pintelaan
9000 Gent
BELGIUM

Carl-Wilhelm Welin
Stockholms Universitet
Inst för Lingvistik
Fack
S-104 05 Stockholm
SWEDEN

Ove Wigertz
Inst f. Medicinsk Teknik
Regionsjukhuset
S-581 85 Linköping
SWEDEN

Gunnar Wijkman
Uppsala Universitet
Box 256
S-751 05 Uppsala
SWEDEN

Friedrich Wingert
Inst. f. Med. Informatik
D-44 Münster
Hüfferstrasse 75
F.R.G.

M. Wolff-Terroine
Institut Gustav Roussy
Service Documentation Scient.
16 bis, Ave. P. Vaillant, Couturier
94 Villejuif
FRANCE

Toshio Yasaka
PL Medical Data Center
Tondabayashi-shi,
Osaka
JAPAN

Sven Öhman
Inst. f. Lingvistik, Box 513
S-751 20 Uppsala, SWEDEN

AUTHOR INDEX